Healing Body *and* Mind

HEALING BODY *AND* MIND

A Critical Issue for Health Care Reform

Roger Kathol, M.D. and Suzanne Gatteau

Foreword by Mary Jane England, M.D.

Praeger Series in Health Psychology
Barbara J. Tinsley, Series Editor

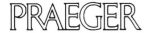

Westport, Connecticut
London

Library of Congress Cataloging-in-Publication Data

Kathol, Roger G.
  Healing body and mind : a critical issue for health care reform / Roger Kathol
and Suzanne Gatteau; foreword by Mary Jane England.
      p.; cm.— (Praeger series in health psychology, ISSN 1543–2211)
  Includes bibliographical references and index.
  ISBN–13: 978–0–275–99201–9 (alk. paper)
  ISBN–10: 0–275–99201–2 (alk. paper)
    1. Mental health services—United States. 2. Health care reform—United
States. I. Gatteau, Suzanne. II. Title. III. Series.
  [DNLM: 1. Mental Health Services—United States. 2. Delivery of Health
Care, Integrated—United States. 3. Health Care Reform—United States. WM
30 K184h 2007]
  RA790.6.K38   2007
  362.1'0425—dc22   2006039615

British Library Cataloguing in Publication Data is available.

Library of Congress Catalog Card Number: 2006039615

ISBN–13: 978–0–275–99201–9
ISBN–10: 0–275–99201–2
ISSN: 1543–2211

First published in 2007

Praeger Publishers, 88 Post Road West, Westport, CT 06881
An imprint of Greenwood Publishing Group, Inc.
www.praeger.com

Printed in the United States of America

The paper used in this book complies with the
Permanent Paper Standard issued by the National
Information Standards Organization (Z39.48–1984).

10   9   8   7   6   5   4   3   2   1

To my patients with concurrent general medical and psychiatric challenges, who have enriched my life and taught me many valuable lessons

CONTENTS

FOREWORD

When I was asked to write the foreword for this book, I had not yet read it. I knew Roger Kathol and respected his work as a clinician, an academic, and a voice for complex patients who need specialized services requiring both medical and psychiatric knowledge. The manuscript of *Healing Body AND Mind* promised to bring to life the recommendations of a major Institute of Medicine (IOM) committee that I had chaired and that had authored, in the Quality Chasm series, a substantial report called *Improving the Quality of Health Care for Mental and Substance Use Conditions.* I was told that the book would carry our published report and our committee to a different level of communication of our findings. I had no idea that the book would be filled with stories of patients and a vision of change.

My first impression, now that I have read *Healing Body AND Mind,* is how readable it is, not only by my scientific and professional colleagues but, more importantly, by those who organize and use health care services—administrators and consumers alike. These pages systematically build the case that mental health and substance-use conditions are an integral part of general medical health. The personal vignettes, or brief narratives about specific patients, caregivers, and their experiences, poignantly illustrate how a separate mental health system retards quality of care and increases health care expense by shifting care and costs for behavioral health to the medical sector. At the current time, mental health and substance-use disorders are largely an afterthought in the larger health reform debate, and this is the discrepancy Kathol's book sets out to communicate and to change.

Not satisfied with just describing the problem that exists at the interface of physical and mental health, *Healing Body AND Mind* walks the reader through a step-by-step example of how health care delivery can be changed. Specifically, and following the IOM recommendations, the change he describes addresses: (1) how patient access to quality mental health and substance-use disorder care can be improved as patients are also treated for their medical illnesses; (2) how health plans can augment support for efficient and effective services in some of their most complex and high-cost members; and (3) how employers and government programs can assist by encouraging the development of medical and behavioral health care work processes that foster a healthier workforce and enrollee population, stimulate greater productivity and less reliance on social services, and lower total health care costs.

Most books of this kind target an audience of professionals in the behavioral health sector because these professionals are the ones who concentrate on ways to improve mental health and substance-use condition treatment. *Healing Body AND Mind,* however, takes two steps beyond such a standard. In addition to communicating to professional practitioners, it provides those who specialize in developing systems for and/or treating patients with general medical conditions with a way to understand the importance of mental health in the context of physical health and the links between the two. Perhaps more significantly, the book also includes consumers in its readership. That is, medical patients with concurrent mental health issues, or vice versa, can read and understand how the system as set up influences their lives and the quality of care they are likely to receive. This empowers them to be a part of the process of necessary change.

Healing Body AND Mind is thus a call to arms not only from health care policy makers but also by those on the front lines: human resource managers, such as Alex; general medical health plan administrators, such as Edward; clinicians, such as Vicki; and patients, such as Kathy, who are affected by poor access to integrated physical and mental health services. At every level, people in the system can become vocal advocates for changing the way that mental health and substance-use disorders are handled. The truth is a simple one: It is only when the voices of patients, administrators, policy makers, and clinicians are all heard in concert and only when they all take steps to create new approaches to care that the system will change.

Healing Body AND Mind closes with a return to the patients described in the first chapter in whom segmented and segregated care led to poor outcomes. The scenarios for these same patients become very different when physical and mental health care are integrated as a part of routine medical practice. Those who choose to read this work will take an adventure into the rationale for making the change, an example of the steps needed to achieve integration, and the outcomes once integrated care is accomplished.

Mary Jane England, M.D.
President, Regis College

PREFACE

By the completion of high school, I had decided that I wanted to become a psychiatrist so that I could apply a medical background to help people suffering with personal and/or emotional problems. It was not until medical school, however, that I found that psychiatry lacked respect from other medical specialties. Its patients were sometimes unpleasant and often severely debilitated. Perhaps more importantly, at the time of my medical school graduation, few used treatments that would predictably change patient outcomes.

Torn by the desire to work with patients suffering psychiatric disturbances, yet wanting to ensure that I was using my talents most effectively by administering treatments that few others could provide, I gravitated toward the scientific discipline of internal medicine, an adult physical health care specialty. Until my senior year in med school, when I took a rotation at the Institute of Psychiatry in London, I had all but decided on a career exclusively in internal medicine. It was during my three months under the tutelage of Professor Michael Sheppard, my houseman Julian Bird, and my senior registrar Robin Murray that I came to understand a revolution was brewing in the field of psychiatry, much like the one that had occurred in internal medicine nearly a century earlier. A growing and dedicated group of psychiatrists were replacing well-intended, but ineffective, approaches to patients with mental health and substance-use disorders with an increasingly accurate system of diagnosis accompanied by treatments with predictably improved outcomes. In effect, psychiatry was going through its own antibiotic and insulin era.

With treatment, the majority of patients with psychiatric illness now could be given a chance to live normal or near normal lives. I wanted to be a part of this important epoch in psychiatric history. At the same time, however, I did not want to surrender the challenge of applying the medical model, wherein accurate diagnosis informed which treatment could be used for the benefit of patients with puzzling physical illnesses. As I debated the direction I would follow, it became apparent that a small but substantial population of patients with psychiatric illness also manifested medical conditions that were hard to address in the psychiatric setting. The reverse was also true for medical patients with psychiatric disorders.

Unexpectedly, I had found an orphan population to which I could devote my professional life that meshed my love of solving the puzzles posed in diagnosing and treating physical illness with my life wish to help patients with mental and substance-use disorders. On the flight back from Europe, I told my wife, Mary, that I was going to do two residencies: internal medicine and psychiatry. With that decision, I began a challenging and rewarding career dedicated to patients with concurrent physical and psychiatric illness.

At the University of Iowa Hospitals and Clinics, with the help and support of a forward-thinking hospital administrator, John Colloton, an adventurous and caring internal medicine department chair, Frank Abboud, and a humorous, dedicated, revolutionist psychiatry chair, George Winokur, I ran what could be arguably described as the best organized inpatient medical psychiatry unit for the care of severely ill patients in the United States, if not the world, for nearly fifteen years. While working in this setting, my appreciation for the frequency and impact that concurrent medical and psychiatric illness had on patients' lives deepened and ignited a passionate concern about the health system that supported their care.

My time at the University of Iowa was a golden period in my career. I treated countless complicated patients, trained dedicated physicians and other health care professionals on how to provide integrated care, and performed research at the interface of physical and mental health. In 1995, while on sabbatical, a time of academic growth but also reflection, I came to the conclusion that I could best contribute to the patients that I cared about and the area of medicine that I practiced by going into medical management consulting with a focus on helping others create treatment-enhancing yet financially solvent integrated physical and behavioral health inpatient and outpatient programs. Few others had my training or experience with these complex and costly inpatients.

Initially, I consulted to hospitals and clinics interested in developing integrated programs in their locations. Because independently managed behavioral health and general medical health plans set up what could accurately be described as a firewall between physical health and behavioral health care, it was a difficult sell. Though hospitals and clinics with integrated programs could reverse the prolonged disease trajectories for some of the most complicated and highest cost patients, they did so at a considerable financial loss. The entrenched provider payment system was not built to support integrated care.

In 2001, in part due to a quirk of fate, I was recruited to help Blue Cross and Blue Shield of Minnesota to integrate general medical and behavioral health business practices at the health plan level. This gave me the opportunity to learn about payment rules that increasingly prevented the coordination of physical and behavioral health care. When Blue Cross and Blue Shield had gone as far as it wanted in its internal transition process, I returned to independent consulting, but now with a concrete understanding of how to accomplish health-improving change.

The experience at Blue Cross allowed me to broaden my consultations to include health plans and employer/government programs. I continued to help clinical programs improve patient care through developing integrated programs and assisted them in developing regional partnerships with health plans and with those who purchased the majority of health care for their constituents. Reimbursement for outcome-changing integrated care became an integral part of my consultation capabilities. This book is intended to summarize what I have learned on a long and eclectic professional path.

Though the subject material is complicated, it is my hope that this book will successfully clarify for people from all backgrounds why it is so difficult to get coordinated care in our current health care environment. Clinicians; hospital, clinic, or health plan administrators; company human resource personnel; government health program negotiators; and the patients, health plan members, or employees who suffer or have suffered with concurrent physical and behavioral health problems will, in one way or another, identify with the complexity and oftentimes bumbling aspects of the health care industry.

I could not have completed this book without the help of my sister Suzanne. She agreed to translate my turgid scientific prose into language suited to a lay audience despite her axe to grind with the U.S. medical system and some of its doctors—which she, with more justification than I like to admit, considers avaricious. I am grateful for her creative input as a writer. I also want to thank my Emmaus brothers for their encouragement, support, and prayers and Les Meyer, Dr. Steven Locke, Fr. Charlie Lachowitzer, and Dr. Keith Folkert for reviewing the book during its development. Their suggestions clearly added to the content and flow.

The greatest thanks and appreciation go to my wife, Mary. She always has been an inspiration and source of support to her family. That has been no less true during the course of this undertaking as many hours of my time, already in short supply, were consumed writing. I am indebted to her for her encouragement, suggestions, and patience.

INTRODUCTION

Health reform debate rages in the United States and in most other countries as health care costs escalate. A significant factor contributing to runaway costs is the segregation of mental and physical health care. Nevertheless, on very few fronts are issues related to the treatment of psychiatric illness in medical patients much more than afterthoughts in discussions about needed change. Behavioral health care, which includes mental and substance-use disorders, consumes only 3 percent to 6 percent of the total health care dollar and exists in a world apart from the rest of medicine. The conventional sentiment among most health policy makers is, "Why even consider physical and behavioral health integration when psychiatric care is an area so peripheral to general medical care, plus the costs associated with it is so limited?" This book explains why decisions about transforming the current health care system must reflect on how the body and mind work in tandem.

Healing Body AND Mind: A Critical Issue for Health Care Reform examines a fragmented health system in which treatment of the mind (mental health) is severed from the body (physical health), resulting in mindless health care. The book unfolds with fictionalized accounts of real patients suffering with concurrent physical and behavioral disorders. They are forced to navigate a health care system that fosters difficult access to segmented and inferior care, which invariably leads to increased health care costs and perpetuated personal suffering and impairment.

The narrative then recounts historical events that reveal staggered, yet parallel, progress in the diagnosis and treatment of physical and psychiatric illness. It highlights the substantial evidence for an interaction between illnesses of the body and the mind, along with the pitfalls of separation in terms of persistent distress from ineffective disease treatment, high costs, illness complications, and lost productivity.

Despite substantial positive reasons to upgrade how behavioral health is treated vis-à-vis physical health, the book explores the many barriers preventing easy evolution to a more beneficial approach to health care. Detailed discussion then takes the reader step-by-step through a health system–level reorganization in which barriers are broken and a process is developed that promotes dramatic improvement in both access to and coordination of clinical care, less complicated handling of mental/substance-use disorder insurance coverage, lower total health care costs, and reduced disease-related impairment due to improved treatment response. The book then returns to the patients from chapter 1 and retells their stories when an integrated approach to health care is available. Healing body *and* mind paints a very different picture.

Because the step-by-step reorganization approach used by Alex, Edward, and Vicki is based on existing models with evidence of outcome improvement, a case is made that transition to an integrated physical and mental/substance-use disorder system, wherein mental health and substance-use disorder care becomes a basic clinical and administrative component of general medical care, can and should be made without delay.

ABBREVIATIONS

AA   Alcoholics Anonymous
ACG   Adjusted clinical groups
ADHD   Attention-deficit/hyperactivity disorder
CAGE   Alcohol dependence screening instrument (C, cut down; A, annoying; G, guilt; E, eye-opener)
CBT   Cognitive behavioral therapy
CDHP   Consumer-driven health plan
CT   Computerized tomography
DBT   Dialectical behavior therapy
DRG   Diagnostic related groups
DSM   *Diagnostic and Statistical Manual of Mental Disorders*
EAP   Employee assistance program
ECT   Electroconvulsive therapy
EEG   Electroencephalogram
ERCP   Endoscopic retrograde cholangiopancreatography
ERISA   Employee Retirement Income Security Act
FDA   Food and Drug Administration
FLOPS   Floating point operations per second
FMLA   Family and Medical Leave Act
GDP   Gross domestic product
GP   General practitioner
HIPAA   Health Insurance Portability and Accountability Act
HMO   Health maintenance organization
HR   Human resources
HSA   Health savings account

IBM	International Business Machines
IPT	Interpersonal psychotherapy
IT	Information technology
K9	Police dog
LTD	Long-term disability
MBHO	Managed behavioral health organization
MCO	Medical care organization
MRI	Magnetic resonance imaging
NMDA	N-methyl-D-aspartate
OHN	Occupational health nurse
PET	Positron-emission tomography
PMI	Psychiatrist for the medically ill
PPO	Preferred provider organization
PST	Problem-solving therapy
SBI	Screening and brief intervention (for alcoholism)
STD	Short-term disability
USC	Unexplained somatic complaint

Chapter 1

"DIS-INTEGRATED" CARE

Our problems are man-made, therefore they may be solved by man.
And man can be as big as he wants. No problem of human destiny is
beyond human beings.[1]

—John F. Kennedy

Three nurses grabbed Nellie, yanked her clothes off and plunged her into a tub of
ice-cold water. After a soap scrub that took the skin off her back and scalp, she
was slammed in the face with a violent splash of the icy water. Three bucketfuls
were poured over her head. Shivering, she climbed out of her bath and was handed
a dirty towel and a thin flannel slip with the label stenciled in back "LUNATIC
ASYLUM, BIH 6."

In 1887, Nellie Bly boldly pushed her way into the executive office of Joseph
Pulitzer, the publisher of the *World,* and changed the course of history.[2] Prepared
to shatter the male domination of his newsroom, Pulitzer offered her a test assignment before officially hiring her to determine if, in fact, she had the mettle for
news reporting. Nellie took the challenge.

The original investigative reporter, Nellie Bly pretended insanity and got herself
committed to New York City's Blackwell Island, an insane asylum for women.
During her 10-day stay, she saw elderly women dragged by the hair and shoved
into closets. She saw girls manacled to one long, thick, iron cable. Sitting on a
hard bench every evening, she ate a slice of stale bread, a saucer of prunes, and a
bowl of tough, stringy meat with blobs of yellow fat in it. Night after night, she
huddled under a ragged blanket, freezing. Nurses in heavy boots strode up and
down between the beds, flashing lanterns into the patients' faces to make sure they
were quiet. "Nobody cared what happened to the insane as long as they were out
of sight," Bly later reported in her newspaper serial "Behind Asylum Bars."

Bly's story ran in September 1887, and it rocked the city. The *World* could not keep up with demand for papers. Outrage swelled. Cries for justice roared, and the scandalous publicity forced city officials to investigate Blackwell Island and other charitable asylums like it. Increased appropriations for competent doctors, good nurses, and scientific research immediately followed. A slow-moving reform toward humane treatment for the insane took root and more than a century later continues to lumber haltingly forward.

What to do with the mentally ill has been an ongoing public debate stretching back several centuries. In the United States, state hospitals provided care, often substandard, for the insane until the introduction of new and effective treatments. With the availability of chlorpromazine and lithium in the mid-1950s, many with serious mental illness were deinstitutionalized and treated in less restrictive environments.

Since then, purportedly in an effort to protect the human rights of mentally ill patients, deinstitutionalization has become accepted policy. It now is a major contributing factor to the current mental health crisis. At present, more than 95 percent of patients, who were previously cared for in state hospitals, have been released. Upon closer examination, the human rights aspect of this gradual exodus from state hospitals has been largely overshadowed by state and federal government attempts to shift costs back and forth to off-load financial responsibility for the mentally ill. We now find that nearly a third of deinstitutionalized seriously mentally ill patients are homeless and half are in and out of jails and prisons, the de facto replacements for state hospitals. Only a sixth are relatively independent.

As troubling as what to do with the mentally ill has been the dispute over what mental illness really is. Historically, society as a whole has assumed that disorders of the mind are separate from disorders of the body. Treatment approaches clearly have reinforced that assumption. People with emotional and behavioral disturbances were, and to a considerable extent still are, considered peripheral to those with so-called real (physical) illness. They are secreted away to separate locations for segregated treatment. In the not too distant past, the domain of medicine focused its efforts exclusively on treatment of illnesses with anatomic and/or physiological abnormalities and regarded the mentally troubled, including substance abusers, as dangerous, untreatable, emotionally weak, and in some cases stained with sin and/or possessed by the devil.

Even as recently as 1975, Anneliese Michel, a 22-year-old German girl, endured twice-weekly exorcisms for nearly a year before she died of malnourishment.[3] According to the Association of Italian Catholic Psychiatrists and Psychologists, today some 500,000 people seek the help of exorcists each year. Now using psychiatric evaluation to distinguish mental illness from possession, the church accepts only a small percentage of these claims as legitimate, but Rome's recently retired chief exorcist and novelist, Fr. Gabriele Amorth, was routinely booked months in advance.[4]

Other familiar and long-popular opinions on mental illness identify a wide range of overused or often misguided psychological defense mechanisms as the cause of psychiatric symptoms. Repression of early childhood experiences is one well-known explanation, but a host of others are hidden in Jungian dream interpretation, existential therapy, and transactional analysis applied to eliminate destructive thought and behavior patterns. Another opinion is shaped by antipsychiatry advocates, such as Scientologists, who deny the existence of mental illness altogether, judging dysfunction of the mind as failure to harness human willpower.

For millennia, the mysterious mind and its relationship to the body has fascinated priests, philosophers, scientists, and doctors. Not until the last half-century, however, has medical science made enormous inroads into our understanding of the genetic, anatomical, physiological, social, and psychological contributors to psychiatric illness as well as of the substantial interaction between mental health/substance-use and physical disorders.

Prior to and even after our understanding of the pathogenesis and the availability of treatment for many now familiar medical illnesses, a portion of patients suffering with epilepsy, rheumatic fever, hyperthyroidism, Huntington's disease, syphilis, and many other medical diseases were treated primarily by *alienists,* the term formerly used to describe psychiatrists. Because these and other medical conditions masqueraded as mental disorders or had psychiatric manifestations, including emotional upheaval, personality change, delusions or hallucinations, and/or abnormal, peculiar bodily movements, the patients often required close observation and behavior control. Many patients with medical disease were, therefore, committed to asylums and treated as other so-called insane patients, often with death as the final outcome from the medical illness causing the psychiatric symptoms.

Today, patients who have medical illnesses that can mimic behavioral disorders have been transferred almost exclusively to the treatment of nonpsychiatrist physicians in non–mental health settings. Early and effective medical treatment usually can prevent the occurrence of psychiatric symptoms. If not prevented, nonpsychiatrist physicians who are willing to incorporate psychiatric treatments along with their medical interventions can effectively reverse mental, along with physical, symptoms.

As importantly, recent studies show that untreated, yet co-occurring, primary psychiatric disorders also require aggressive intervention in those with physical illness because they are associated with worse clinical, functional, and economic outcomes. Concurrent primary psychiatric disorders merely can be coincidental to general medical disorders or can be caused by them. For instance, schizophrenia, anxiety disorder, substance abuse, bipolar or unipolar depression, autism, eating disorders, cognitive impairment, and so forth are frequently seen in those with general medical illness.

Alternatively, medical conditions may be the direct result of a psychiatric illness or its treatment. Gunshot wounds or intoxications in suicidal patients, obesity and diabetes in patients taking some of the new antipsychotic medications, and physician-created adverse events due to unnecessary medical tests or medications in somatizing patients, with or without depression or anxiety, represent several examples of this type of association.

Scientifically, we are on the cusp of dramatic improvements in the treatment of patients who have general medical and psychiatric illnesses occurring at the same time (comorbid illness). Every year, medical illnesses and medications are added to the list of those associated with the development of behavioral symptoms. To the extent that early identification of the offending general medical condition or medication is made, significant mental health impairment often can be prevented, or at least attenuated, by effective treatment. Conversely, with the new techniques available to uncover brain abnormalities and to identify psychiatric syndromes, it is now possible to predictably uncover and reverse emotional suffering and aberrant behaviors and to lower costs by utilizing advances in biological and psychological treatments both for patients with mental health/substance-use disorders alone or for those with concurrent physical illness.

Unfortunately, the opportunity to move forward with effective clinical approaches to care for patients with interacting general medical and behavioral health disorders is stymied by a health system that *prevents* early identification of concurrent illness and the coordination of psychiatric and nonpsychiatric services. With collaborative support and interventions from psychiatrists and other behavioral health professionals, the ability of nonpsychiatrist physicians to uncover and effectively treat patients with psychological disorders can be greatly enhanced.

The severed alliance between physical and mental health/substance-use disorder specialists as a result of independently managed general medical and psychiatric care, however, frustrates success. As a result, patients with behavioral disorders use twice as many total health care services yet have worse general medical and psychiatric outcomes and are less productive at work.[5] They also account for the lion's share of disability payments.

Operations in hospitals and clinics in today's health care system are driven by autonomous general medical and behavioral health business practices that require or encourage separate clinician networks, segregated and poorly coordinated physical and mental health settings for the same patients, discrepant service access approval processes, and inequitable payment. These business practices necessarily impede communication between health providers and generate higher health-related costs, especially medical, for patients with unaddressed psychiatric illness and ineffectively treated physical conditions.

The high cost of treating these patients, coupled with the dismal success of the nonintegrated treatment given, logically would predict an aggressive move toward training nonpsychiatrist physicians to identify and treat patients with concurrent physical and psychiatric illness, with or without the help of their behavioral health colleagues. Not so. Most medical health practitioners do not realize the impact that concurrent illness has on clinical, functional, and economic outcomes for their patients. Further, they have little reason to look into behavioral health issues because they already are overwhelmed with tasks in their own discipline.

Care for psychologically distressed patients remains in the outer realm of the general medical domain. Likewise, physical health questions rarely are asked in the mental health/substance-use disorder setting. Hospitals maintain rigid separation of medical and psychiatry units. Insurance companies write plans disregarding the potential mind-body complexity of comorbid general medical and psychiatric illnesses and their treatment. This so-called mindless health care approach to healing continues to cripple the progress of a technological medical boon. Patients, health providers, employers, human services departments, and insurance companies all share the strife of one additional component of an already anemic health care system.

In the twenty-first century, Nellie Bly probably would not encounter old ladies stuffed into closets at an insane asylum. Instead, she would listen curiously, pen poised, to people like Eva, Mohammed, and scores of other patients who are forced to navigate a cumbersome, costly, and ineffectual health care system.

* * *

Eva rolled over, turned off the alarm clock, and sat on the edge of the bed, her swollen feet tingling on the oak floor. Already she was exhausted. She woke up her two children and put a box of cereal on the kitchen table for their breakfast. A headache teased at her temples, and she felt woozy, like she had a bad hangover. She held the cell phone, fingers itching to punch in the office number to report another sick day, but resisted the impulse. Her absences doubled her coworkers' workload, and their resentment was palpable.

In the shower, Eva steadied herself against the tile, and tears mingled with soapsuds ran down her cheeks. Simply, Eva had no energy. Dishes piled up in the sink, empty bags of cookies gathered on tabletops, and newspapers yellowed on the front doorstep. Even the small task of tucking in her children at night was a supreme effort. The vibrant dynamo she once had been was now a 43-year-old absentee, avoiding social interaction and personal responsibility.

An information technology (IT) specialist, Eva was a stellar performer for five of the seven years of her employment with Information Systems. She was active in volunteer programs and divisional functions, a regular at the company's exercise facility, and sparkled with enthusiasm at social events. During the last two years, her performance had dramatically declined and her lack of participation was conspicuous. More and more often, the human resources (HR) department logged in Eva's sick days. "I'm just tired," she told her friends.

Initially, Eva's primary care doctor attributed her decline to an inability to control her chronic diabetes, but Eva claimed to be following diet, exercise, and insulin routines as she always had. Nevertheless, her glucose was curiously more often elevated than controlled. Twice within the past year she had been hospitalized with dangerously high blood sugar levels that necessitated an insulin pump.

A phone call from Eva's behavioral health plan network counselor, whom she had been seeing on her own since her recent divorce, alerted her doctor that something other than diabetes might be contributing to the decline. According to the counselor, Eva had experienced the onset of recurrent major depression nine months ago, twenty years after her first episode. The counselor had been working, unsuccessfully, with her on family issues.

Based on this new information, her doctor gave her a prescription for Prozac with a follow-up appointment six weeks later. Unfortunately, and unknown to him, she took the medication for only two weeks because the pills disturbed her sleep. She also stopped seeing her counselor because the sessions, after exceeding her health plan's annual limit, had become her sole financial responsibility. Symptomatic of depression, Eva's hopelessness, lack of concentration, and inactivity disengaged her motivation to take the necessary steps to control her diabetes. She did not check her glucose levels, ate indiscriminately, and stopped exercising, which compounded the depression and accelerated diabetic sensory loss and vision problems.

The poorly controlled diabetes-depression combination eventually compelled Eva's doctor to recommend short-term disability until her diabetes stabilized. While her diabetic foot ulcer threatened to turn into gangrene, his efforts at stabilization were futile. He did not know that Eva was not routinely taking her medication for depression and would never know. She was too embarrassed to tell him how lax she had become.

Eva's situation is typical of chronic, complex medical conditions. For nearly a year, her doctor attributed deterioration in her diabetes to physiological changes and treated her, at enormous medical cost, for uncontrolled diabetes. After being alerted by her counselor, he realized depression was undermining Eva's ability to adhere to her medical treatment and prescribed accordingly. Even then, the lack of coordination with Eva's counselor, limits in Eva's behavioral health benefits, and less than honest information from Eva left her doctor with little chance of improving Eva's health.

* * *

Mohammed hurled his grammar book across the room and, ranting insults at his mother, bolted out the backdoor. "I hate you!" he yelled. Mrs. Zar stood on the deck wringing her hands, frustrated and hopeless. Even though he scored highly on national tests, Mohammed's grades had plummeted steadily over the past months. Notes from his teacher were frequently mailed home reporting temper tantrums, missed homework assignments, class disruption, and discipline problems. At home, he either sulked or ignited chaos. More often he could not sleep and roamed the house playing inappropriate practical jokes on his siblings or channel surfing until exhaustion knocked him out. His mother walked on eggshells, and the civility between Mohammed and his dad was tenuous.

Mohammed's mother watched her troubled 11-year-old sprint down the street with the fury of a forest fire until he disappeared, then she called their pediatrician. Later that week, Dr. John took Mohammed's history and conducted a physical examination. He obtained a blood count, thyroid and glucose levels, and even a brain wave test (electroencephalogram, or EEG). When the tests came back normal, the doctor suspected Mohammed may suffer from attention-deficit/hyperactivity disorder, commonly known as ADHD, and urged his mother to make an appointment with a child psychiatrist who could make a definitive diagnosis.

Because health insurance plans vary widely, each with its own behavioral health subcontractors, Dr. John could not give Mrs. Zar a personal referral. Instead, he showed her how to find the 800-number for behavioral health providers on the back of her insurance card. The 800-number operator gave Mrs. Zar three child psychiatrists' numbers, none of whom were taking new patients. She called the phone bank again and was given another three names. On the fifth try, she found a doctor who could fit Mohammed into his schedule in five months. In the meantime, Mohammed's disruptive, nonproductive behavior escalated, and Dr. John prescribed the stimulant Ritalin (methylphenidate) to ease the turmoil in the interim.

At the appointment, an overbooked Dr. Jerry did a short evaluation on Mohammed, noting a family history of bipolar disorder. When asked about the effectiveness of the stimulant that Dr. John had prescribed, Mrs. Zar reported "good weeks and bad weeks." Dr. Jerry made adjustments in the meds and scheduled a follow-up appointment. Dr. Jerry sent the examination report to Dr. John, indicating a concern about bipolar illness only after he was assured that a release had been signed. The Health Insurance Portability and Accountability Act (HIPAA) privacy rules made him extracautious, even though he knew that it was important for Dr. John to have the results of Mohammed's evaluation. Frustrated by the curt, cursory examination, Mrs. Zar canceled their timely follow-up with Dr. Jerry.

As time went on, Mohammed's earlier control deteriorated. His anger attacks intensified, and he blamed his teachers and parents. He morphed into the playground bully, making sexually indiscreet innuendos and threats both to his classmates and to school employees. With Mohammed spinning out of control, Mrs. Zar tried to schedule an emergency appointment with Dr. Jerry again and, failing, relied on the independent advice of her pediatrician Dr. John to juggle the meds in an effort to reverse Mohammed's destructive ADHD behaviors. Dr. John had never started mood stabilizers himself and was reluctant to change the stimulants or push the dosage for fear of medical and/or legal repercussion. "Give it time," he said. "He's a teenager; he'll grow out of this."

Mohammed's grades hit rock bottom; school suspensions were commonplace and expulsion imminent. Mrs. Zar, without resource or connection, tried to get her son enrolled in a school for at-risk children. She was in the process of setting this up when Mohammed, who now saw himself as a failure, attempted suicide by swallowing all the pills from nearly a full bottle of Tylenol in the medicine cabinet. Though Mohammed had gone to bed as if nothing had happened, Mrs. Zar luckily found the empty bottle in the bathroom wastebasket. Tylenol does not kill immediately like other medications. The victim dies slowly, weeks later, of liver failure.

* * *

Keith, Coastal Care medical director, and his staff routinely isolate and review the small segment of his company's subscriber population that uses the majority of medical benefits. Margie's case came to his attention when Susan, a Coastal Care medical case manager, questioned whether to approve another surgery that Margie was requesting.

Keith manipulated the keyboard, Ctrl PgDn, and Subscriber #A-77754 appeared on the monitor screen.

Benefits paid out: 2005/$47,000—2006/$93,000

Subscriber: 33-year-old female, married, one child.

"Primary" complaints in 2005 and 2006 included: abdominal pain, weakness, bloating, and food sensitivities.

He recognized Margie's record immediately.

Margie's intestinal problems began in her late teens with intermittent stomachaches that bottles of Pepto-Bismol did not cure. Dr. Jane, Margie's family pediatrician, never could diagnose for certain what caused the severe abdominal complaints that often landed Margie in the emergency room and occasionally into the hospital. At Margie's mother's insistence, Dr. Jane aggressively evaluated symptoms until Margie left for college.

Eventually, Margie's abdominal complaints took second fiddle to headaches, limb weakness, spastic neck, urinary pain, and many sundry afflictions. Her name appeared often on many doctors' office rosters. Marriage and childbirth increased the frequency of doctor appointments, and when one of the doctors pointed out that the pressure of motherhood might be the root of her troubles, she crossed him off her list of trustworthy doctors.

Between 2003 and 2005, Keith noted that Margie had seen at least nine different local community primary care physicians and four stomach specialists. X-ray technicians at several hospitals knew Margie on a first-name basis. Out of frustration, a stomach specialist had persuaded a surgeon colleague to perform an exploratory abdominal procedure, not realizing that a similar operation by a general practitioner had turned up nothing several years before.

By 2005, Margie had run out of doctors in her local community and was now traveling several hundred miles to see specialists at a world-renowned academic medical center. Once admitted and housed in a private room, Margie refused to release prior medical information to her new doctors because she wanted a "fresh look" without bias. Because Margie was determined to call her own shots and was adequately insured through her husband's large manufacturing company, the specialists had no recourse but to cater to her demands.

An initial noninvasive evaluation revealed no abnormalities in Margie's health condition. Nonspecific treatment, however, even with some of the newest antireflux, antigas, and antispasmodics, failed to mitigate her stomach complaints for longer than several weeks. More aggressive X-rays, scopings, angiograms, biopsies, and titers ensued during the next 12 months, some during hospitalizations of a week or more. In addition to intestine-focused evaluations, many other minor complaints were evaluated and/or treated. Margie had at least thirty different medications in her pill basket, a third that she used regularly.

Only after the intestinal specialists and the many medical and surgical consultants had exhausted options and work-ups, another belly exploration was proposed. When this proposal came to the attention of Susan, Margie's case manager, because of Margie's consistently high annual claims, Keith got involved. Keith, who had the benefit of claims data, immediately noticed that Margie was going through her third complete evaluation for abdominal complaints in the past 10 years. In addition, the records showed numerous doctor involvements tallying 15 major and minor procedures, 70-plus prescriptions, and many tests performed and repeated, seemingly indiscriminately.

Keith knew that he should not approve another procedure, but what recourse did he have? She was being seen by some of the best physicians in the country.

They were recommending something Keith knew was very costly and would have a low yield, but his hands were tied. He reluctantly approved.

* * *

For the last half-hour, Tommy had listened to Alvin's breathing get progressively more labored, the wheezing louder, but he knew better than to ask to take over at the wheel. Tommy remembered other times when the breathing spells had happened on their route. Alvin had been too proud and too stubborn to surrender control of the 20-ton waste management truck. This time, Tommy kicked back, kept his mouth shut, and hoped for a smooth ride back to the plant. Ten minutes later, Alvin made a right turn onto a side street and parked the rig. Agitated, he fumbled for his cell phone.

"What gives?" Tommy asked.

"Call 911, man. I can't get a breath."

In the ambulance, the medics restored Alvin's breathing with oxygen, epinephrine, and bronchodilators. Later at the hospital ER, they hooked him up to an intravenous line and adjusted the medications. Gradually, Alvin's air passages opened up, and his primary care physician, Dr. Julie, admitted him for observation and stabilization.

This was not out of the ordinary for Alvin. A long history of asthma complicated by anxiety attacks and depression rendered Alvin an unreliable employee with chronic illness. Over the past three years, he averaged three months of sick leave annually at a substantial cost to the company in man-hours as well as to the insurance companies responsible for his health care expenditures. His routine absences resulted in decreased company productivity, extravagant overtime expenses, and havoc in route schedule adjustments.

Karen, the health risk manager for National Waste Management, was well aware of Alvin's crises. As overseer of employees' health conditions, she wondered why Alvin's poor health resisted improvement. Alvin had access to many assistance services through the company's employee benefits program, a combination of services that she thought would assure maximum health for its employees and would, in turn, optimize employee productivity. She presumed that the company's disease management program with AdvancedDM had detailed the necessary information to Alvin regarding his asthma and that Alvin had been given an impressive three-color, professionally prepared packet describing the available asthma treatments with names and numbers of providers in the company's network.

Karen also knew that Sophie, the company's occupational health nurse, occasionally had talked with Alvin about his health issues, but privacy matters had prevented Sophie sharing with Karen critical information that could have facilitated a better outcome for both Alvin and National Waste Management. Sophie knew that Alvin's asthma was complicated by depression and anxiety. Early in her assessment, she had considered referring Alvin to the employee assistance program (EAP). Her previous experience with the company's EAP, though, indicated that their involvement was limited to a pep talk with no real involvement, plus the enrollment process was cumbersome. She, like Karen, was under the impression that Alvin had been working with AdvancedDM.

Dr. Julie, Alvin's primary care physician, though not well versed on the dynamics or connection between asthma, anxiety, and depression, did understand that Alvin's physiological symptoms were exacerbated by his mental state. She prescribed alprazolam to control his anxiety attacks, but Alvin had told her "I'm no mental freak" and refused to take the medication. After one visit to the mental health clinic, he never went back. Just having his car parked in their lot embarrassed him.

The disability management team got involved when Alvin's absences exceeded the disability guidelines for time off needed to control asthma. After reviewing the most recent claim documenting another acute asthma attack, short-term disability was once again approved. Their report alerted Karen to a serious flaw in managing Alvin's situation, but she was stumped as to where to pinpoint the problem.

The plethora of assembled health managers, available at no cost to Alvin to keep him healthy and productive, were adept at meeting the letter of their health management responsibilities but inept at helping Alvin manage his asthma, anxiety, and depression. Blame can be placed on no one arm of the system. Despite Karen's dedication and effort on behalf of the employees she represented, all participated in the poor outcome of Alvin's health crisis, including Alvin.

The asthma brochure the disease management team gave him five years ago had never been opened. With an eighth-grade education, he did not have the patience or motivation to wade through a bunch of stuff he did not understand. He had not taken the time to discuss with professionals the difference between an anxiety attack and an asthma attack. As a result, many times he put his health in jeopardy by not seeking measures early enough to avoid an expensive ambulance ride to a hospital emergency room and the customary admission.

When he was feeling good, he figured he was cured. Feeling cured, he quit taking his meds and left the inhaler at home. Because no one followed up on Alvin's mismanagement of his own health until it reached a crisis level, his chronic condition prevailed.

* * *

Ellen, the chief executive officer (CEO); Rachel, her chief financial officer (CFO); and Andrew, the chief medical officer (CMO) at Mercy Hospital met regularly to review high-service-use cases that far outstripped their diagnostic related group (DRG—to be explained later) insurance reimbursement. The goal of their meeting was ostensibly to determine how to improve outcomes and reduce lengths of stay for patients with complex illness, but the unspoken objective was to prevent unnecessary financial loss from patient cost outliers, meaning those for whom the cost of treatment exceeds reimbursement. Because Mercy was only a small 150-bed community hospital, they could not afford to lose revenue.

Ellen pulled an itemized bill on Mrs. Abraham from a list of admissions during the prior month. She had a recent 22-day stay with a discharge diagnosis of stomach ulcer complicated by a dislocated shoulder. Mrs. Abraham had spent 8 days in the intensive care unit (ICU) and 12 on a general medicine unit, yet the discharge diagnoses were for conditions that did not typically require admission. The mean length of stay for small stomach ulcer was still only four days. Why Mrs. Abraham had stayed so long and required ICU care was a question that needed an answer.

A resident at Samaritan Senior Center, Mrs. Abraham was a 77-year-old lady, weighing in at 103 pounds. During the week before she arrived at the emergency room by ambulance, she had become increasingly confused and combative. Her geriatrician described her as a "fragile senior citizen." He recorded that "it didn't take much to set her off." His last clinical note, sent with her from the assisted-living facility, confirmed that she had been on Aricept (donepezil), a memory-preserving medication, for several years as a treatment for midstage dementia.

Other than this, Mrs. Abraham, previously very athletic, was remarkably healthy. She had an allergy to sulfa medications, first noted when she was treated for a kidney infection years earlier. Also, from time to time, she complained of an old shoulder injury from a skiing accident. Cancer and emphysema were noted in her family history. Aricept was her only medication. Her last admission had been five years ago for pneumonia associated with the flu. Mrs. Abraham would have been transferred by ambulance to a stand-alone psychiatric hospital with a geriatric unit except that she had an unexplained low blood count.

The first day in the hospital was a challenge for doctors and nursing staff. Mrs. Abraham refused blood tests and other medical assistance. She slapped and pushed one nurse who she thought was trying to poison her by giving her a pill to calm her down. She refused to let the doctor do more than get vitals, listen to her chest, and poke on her stomach. A stool sample from a messy bed tested positive for trace blood but did not show evidence of active bleeding; however, Mrs. Abraham refused abdominal X-rays and certainly would not let anyone put a tube down her mouth (endoscope) to look for ulcers. In hopes that she would calm down with time, she was put in soft restraints to protect her from falling out of bed and then left alone. This was when Mrs. Abraham began yelling incessantly for help—day and night.

By the fourth day of hospitalization, both a psychiatric consultation and a cognitive assessment by a neuropsychologist had been obtained. Both agreed that Mrs. Abraham was delirious, that is, confused, likely due to some unrecognized physical illness.

The psychiatrist suggested intravenous haloperidol be given because it had quicker action and higher response rates for delirious behavior than the atypical antipsychotic suppositories and intramuscular injections that Mrs. Abraham's doctors were using. The doctors, however, were reluctant to follow the psychiatrist's advice because they were unfamiliar with the use of intravenous haloperidol administration.

That evening, the staff realized that restraints without constant observation and failure to follow the psychiatrist's suggestion had been a mistake. Having escaped from one of her restraints, Mrs. Abraham was found dangling from the side of her bed by the arm that remained restrained. Fortunately, that restraint had been short enough that Mrs. Abraham had not hit her head on the floor, but she had dislocated her arm.

With the aide of an orthopedic surgeon, the arm was popped back into place, but Mrs. Abraham then required a sling and pain medications in addition to the medications being used to attempt to control her behavior. This only increased her confusion and combativeness. The general medical unit was already short-staffed and there were no qualified nurse sitters available for such a disabled and combative patient. Plus, the nursing staff was frazzled with Mrs. Abraham's constant yelling. Finally, she was transferred to the intensive care unit, which periodically happened when sick delirious patients could not be controlled. Members of her family, who lived in a neighboring state, were notified. Upon their arrival, they were stunned by their mother's condition.

In the ICU, Mrs. Abraham continued to be impervious to the tranquilizing medications. For 24 hours while in a full-body restraint, attempts were made to control her thrashing and yelling with escalating doses of medications for pain and confusion. Shots in the buttocks came more frequently but to little avail. She went back and forth from oversedated to combative. Intravenous haloperidol remained outside the comfort zone for Mrs. Abraham's ICU doctors, even with continuous cardiac monitors and 24-hour nurse coverage.

An intravenous line was inserted to provide adequate food and fluid requirements, and a bladder catheter kept track of fluid balance. More than a week after Mrs. Abraham's admission, a decision was finally made to put her under anesthesia so the doctors could look at the stomach through an endoscope. Sure enough, there was a small ulcer eating at her stomach. Positive for *Helicobacter pylori,* bacteria now shown to cause ulcers, she was immediately placed on an antibiotic cocktail, a stomach acid suppressor, and a stomach-lining protector. Additional days in the ICU were required before the delirium improved and the medical conditions stabilized.

When Mrs. Abraham was finally considered stable enough to return to the general medical unit, she still required soft restraints but this time with a 24-hour sitter to make sure she sustained no further injuries. Over the next week, she progressively returned to her forgetful, yet cooperative self. She was discharged to a nursing home for convalescence and rehabilitation before she could return to her assisted-living facility. Dumbfounded that a small stomach ulcer could be so devastating, her children learned from the doctor that similar situations in the elderly had occurred many times before.

After reviewing the hospital stay, Ellen, Rachel, and Andrew concluded that there was nothing their staff could have done to change the course of the hospital stay. The main oversight from their standpoint was not ordering a sitter early during the admission. The medical staff, however, could not be faulted for this because the executive trio themselves had put out a memorandum not more than a month before encouraging judicious and conservative use of constant nursing observation. A recent audit had shown that 24-hour observation nurse extras accounted for nearly a quarter-million dollars in unreimbursed expense for the hospital.

The little community hospital had no choice but to absorb the loss of $45,900 ($51,500 actual cost of hospital stay minus the $5,600 Medicare DRG reimbursement rate for their hospital) for Mrs. Abraham's care as a cost of doing business.

* * *

Harry is 38 and has worked on the assembly line at Capitol Industries for 13 years. He has always been a responsible and energetic employee, husband, and father. With ruddy cheeks and an easy laugh, he is a welcomed guest everywhere he goes. "Drinks all around," he yells out to the bartender. The table crowds with friends, and Harry sucks down gin and tonics while his stories weave and laughter tumbles.

When morning comes, Harry chews a handful of Tums and prods at the point of pain in his gut. "An ulcer," the doc had said. "Cut back on the alcohol." And Harry had cut back. Instead of unwinding with a six-pack after work, he limited himself to three beers a night on weekdays. On weekends he no longer mixed his alcohols, choosing to make it either a beer weekend or a gin weekend, and during the six weeks of Lent he had given up hard liquor altogether. Nevertheless, on Monday mornings indigestion was common. His perpetual stomach bloat would balloon and his energy plummeted.

The morning after the preseason opener for the Redskins, Harry hugged the toilet and coughed up blood. His wife rushed him to the emergency room, where they forced a tube down his throat to take pictures of his digestive tract. Then they gave him two units of blood. Later that afternoon, Dr. Anita, the gastrointestinal doctor assigned to his case, diagnosed bleeding esophageal varices. She explained that blocked drainage from a scarred liver had severely expanded the blood vessels in his esophagus. The vomiting had irritated them enough that one of the vessels sprang a leak. His condition was more dangerous than ulcers because the bleeding could be heavy and hard to stop. "He had been lucky," she reported.

Ten days later, awaiting discharge from the hospital, Dr. Ken, Harry's primary care physician, asked to speak with Harry, his wife, and any other family members Harry wished to include. Sitting in the sterile hospital room, flower bouquets wilting on the window ledge, Dr. Ken told the assembled family that a needle biopsy confirmed that Harry's liver showed end-stage cirrhosis. The prognosis was blunt. If Harry intended to live long enough to see his sons graduate from high school, he would have to quit drinking and put his name on the list for a liver transplant.

Unlike many alcoholics, Harry had rarely missed a day of work. He was a so-called happy drunk, a good provider, and a wonderful man. An active mentor in Boy Scouts and junior varsity football and treasurer of the Kiwanis Club, he was a pillar of the community. Though occasionally his slurred speech and rowdy behavior embarrassed his family and unsettled his associates, nobody made a big deal about it. He deserved to have one little vice, did he not?

Unfortunately, Harry's one little vice was his death warrant. Even though Dr. Ken had repeatedly told Harry his ballooning belly, sallow complexion, easy bruising, increasing fatigue, and enlarged breasts were all serious warning signs, Harry had ignored them, and now his options were limited.

Masking snowballing anxiety, he said, "So doc, bottom line, it's a play-you-pay kind of situation I got here?"

"Bottom line, that's the situation, Harry."

Dr. Ken arranged an assessment with the liver transplant service, and after reviewing Harry's record, the administrator reported that Harry would have to have chemical dependency treatment before requesting a liver transplant. Further, before authorizing the several-hundred-thousand-dollar operation, they would need certification from the facility that Harry had completed the program and been sober for at least six months. The cost for the required 28-day inpatient alcohol treatment was $22,200 with the extended six-week outpatient program and consolidating gains another $5,300. Dr. Ken assured Harry that many health plans covered this service, and he felt confident that Harry's plan would pick up the tab.

Capitol Industries offered a flexible health plan to their employees, giving each employee a choice of what services they wanted covered by insurance. Ten years ago, with the expense of three young children and a new house on his shoulders, Harry decided to opt out of a number of available benefits he felt were not applicable to his family's needs. Regrettably for Harry, one of the benefits he dropped was chemical dependence treatment, and once dropped, he could not add it.

Harry and his wife's combined salaries provided a comfortable lifestyle for their family. They tucked away enough annual savings for a camping trip to the Rockies or a necessary home improvement project. Recently, they had started a purse to help with their sons' college educations. Once in awhile, they earmarked a dollar here, a dollar there, hoping to one day upgrade their personal computer.

To come up with $27,500 was like asking for the moon.

Harry argued fiercely with the health plan administrator. How could he have known he would need alcoholism treatment? The administrator, though sympathetic, explained that the whole purpose of insurance was to prepare for the unexpected, and he was sorry, but he could not bend the rules. The expense was Harry's alone, and his life depended on it.

* * *

Each of these cases provides examples of a broken system and illustrates how segregation of general medical and behavioral health care leads to less than satisfactory care and worse health outcomes.

- Eva's story describes poor coordination between health providers in addressing the complexity of her diabetes and depression.
- Mohammed's struggle highlights the communication gaps that exist between pediatricians and those involved in behavioral health support for children, a particularly difficult area due to the shortages of child psychiatrists.
- Margie represents the 10 percent of health care users who populate the cost outlier category and consume more than two-thirds of the health care dollar. This group of patients drives medical plan directors, like Keith, to consume extraordinary amounts of Mylanta while trying to responsibly divvy out limited medical resources for undiagnosed patients presenting unexplained somatic complaints.
- Alvin, sensitive to the stigma of mental illness, is caught up in a maze of well-intended but disjointed health programs that fail on every level to communicate with him.
- Mrs. Abraham's simple stomach ulcer remained undiagnosed for nearly a week because her doctors could not control her delirious behavior enough to diagnose the underlying cause. In the meantime, she sustained an unnecessary complication

that led to an extended hospital stay. With no recourse, the hospital was responsible for much of the cost.

- Harry's conundrum reflects the convoluted bias and inconsistencies of health insurance coverage, a hotbed of controversy that will be discussed in detail in later chapters.

Although there are numerous problems within the U.S. and other worldwide health systems, fragmented carved-out behavioral health care from general medical services contributes significantly to ineffective health care. Poor clinical outcomes and higher health care costs are the legacy of an approach to mindless healing. Though the challenges and barriers facing most health systems are intimidating, they are not without solutions. Traveling from the early history of medicine to modern-day medical marvels, this book will explore how the rewards of integrating general medical and behavioral health far outweigh the effort and costs required to make the transition.

Chapter 2

HEALTH PROGRESS

The most powerful drive in the ascent of man is his pleasure in his own skill. He loves to do what he does well and, having done well, he loves to do it better.[1]

—Jacob Bronowski

HISTORICAL OVERVIEW

A conclave of doctors did not one day sit in a boardroom and decide psychiatry must become a specialty of medicine. There was no job description or study guide. Rather, a few renegade doctors, horrified by the brutality they witnessed in care institutions for the insane, broke rank and actively sought more scientific explanations and better treatment for those with mental illness.

The branch of medicine dedicated to improving the identification and treatment of mental illness and substance abuse that is in place today evolved ever so slowly over millennia. Ancient Sanskrit records, circa 1400 B.C., show that physicians in India established shelters for mentally ill persons. Plato in 400 B.C. wrote about melancholia and described manic states, suggesting in both instances that base emotions clamored to overwhelm the rational soul. Archeologists researching preindustrial groups have cataloged colorful and fascinating evidence of Native American shaman ceremonies that were performed to expel evil spirits and restore the lost soul.

The Swiss anatomist Felix Plater spent years studying so-called mad persons, many of whom he found imprisoned in dungeons as suspected witches during the Inquisition. Plater concluded then that mad persons suffered from alienation because their illness separated them from their true selves. Because the alienation theory was popular in its day, the term stuck, and doctors specializing in the treatment of the insane were originally known as alienists.

In 1329 in London, St. Mary's Priory opened a home for the needy—a few homeless, a few lepers. In time, the shelter was taken over by the Crown and became the city hospital for the mentally ill, eventually to include the criminally insane as well. London's Bethlem Royal Hospital, later shortened to madhouse or Bedlam, was one of the original asylums for the deranged. Thousands and thousands of odiously described accounts attest to the inhumane treatment that went on behind closed gates. In Shakespeare-speak, *bedlam* connoted noise and disorder, an apt description for a place that housed shrieking half-naked inmates lying on straw with their legs chained to crude blocks of wood. On Sunday afternoons for the price of a penny, London citizens were invited to gawk and jeer at the lunatics on display (Figure 2.1).[2] In 1815, Bedlam collected £400 in pennies from some 96,000 visitors.

In 1793, the French alienist Philippe Pinel (considered by some to be the father of psychiatry), hoping to generate a self-reparative process, introduced moral treatment for the insane.[3] He changed the term *lunatic* to *patient,* banished the use of chains, and demanded that filthy cells be cleaned. Pinel reported

Figure 2.1 Asylum as entertainment.
William Hogarth's Plate 8 of *A Rake's Progress,* **created in 1763, depicts Bedlam as a place of entertainment for the well-dressed noble ladies shown in the background.**

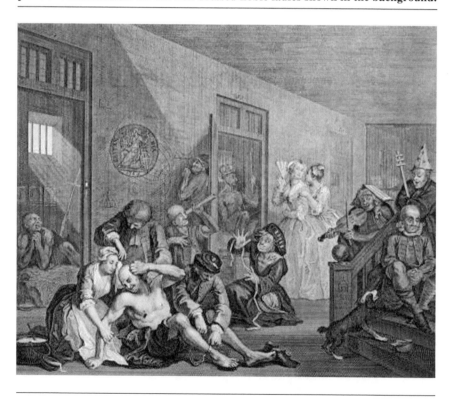

to alarmed madhouse philanthropists and directors that disturbed patients could benefit from kind and imaginative treatment. Though a worthy endeavor, cost factors and lack of demonstrable clinical improvement interfered as a growing number of patients sought assistance. Building suitable facilities and staffing the asylums to provide restorative care became prohibitive and, as evidenced in Nellie Bly's 1887 account, Dr. Pinel's forward-thinking approach slipped back to custodial care.

It is important to put the slow but methodical advances in psychiatric treatment into perspective by comparing them to advances in other medical disciplines. Extensive early progress in medicine occurred nearly a century before advances were made in psychiatry, but the momentum for both was pockmarked with misadventure. As far back as when Leonardo da Vinci was stealing cadavers in order to study human anatomy, the science of healing has been an exercise of trial and error.

Early History of Medical Treatment

The familiar blood-red-striped barbershop pole is thought to have its origin in the barber-surgeon. When the local medicine woman's bag of bat guano failed to promote wound healing, the neighborhood barber intervened. Before antibiotics, narcotics, and anesthesia made the scene, deep swigs of whiskey cushioned the bite of the saw as infected limbs were amputated in an attempt to save lives. Even then, death from infection was typical because hands and surgical instruments were not sterilized.

It was only after Ignaz Semmelweis, an obstetrician in Budapest, introduced sterile technique in 1848 that death from surgery-related infection plummeted.[4] Many mothers were dying within a week or two after giving birth from a disease doctors called childbed fever or the curse of Eve. Deaths from puerperal fever (as it is known today) were far more common in the obstetric ward where medical students delivered babies directly after coming from the dissecting or autopsy rooms than in the ward run by midwives who were careful about cleanliness. This piqued Semmelweis's interest. After applying brilliant fact-finding and analysis, he concluded that infected particles left on the medical students' unwashed hands and surgical tools were the source of the deadly infections. As a result, he instituted the use of lime chloride for hand and instrument washing between surgeries.

Despite tabulating a remarkable reduction in the death rate from puerperal fever in new mothers, Dr. Semmelweis met forceful opposition, and the director of the hospital made sure the obstetrician's contract was not extended. The majority of his colleagues took exception to the idea that the hands of a doctor could be unclean. Nowadays, we take sterile technique for granted, but it took decades for the medical profession to adopt this simple lifesaving procedure.

Earlier, a similar bull-headed reaction to empirical data had crystallized around bleeding, a treatment used for millennia in a wide range of illnesses. Attesting to the level of sophistication the treatment had attained, numerous calendars recovered from the medieval era meticulously designate the best astrological times for bloodletting. Needless to say, when Dr. P.C.A. Louis published that there was no benefit from bloodletting in his book *Researches on the Effects of Bloodletting in Some Inflammatory Diseases* in 1836, he was not a popular guy.[5]

Dr. Louis ended up apologizing for his findings, and it took another 20 years of proof and reproof to convince physicians not to use the procedure in their clinical practice. His apology saved him his job. Semmelweis, who did not proffer an apology, met only ridicule and was not vindicated until Louis Pasteur identified the Hungarian's theory of contagion in 1879, 14 years after Semmelweis's death.

Ample present-day examples of medical interventions thought to be of value have proved otherwise. Scandal-ridden and costly bone marrow transplantation, used as a treatment to cure advanced breast cancer in the mid-1990s, eventually was found to lead to higher mortality and is no longer a suggested option. An article in the *New England Journal of Medicine* in 2002 reported that arthroscopic knee lavage (washing out the knee space) and debridement (cleaning the rough edges of knee structures) for osteoarthritis (degenerative joint disease) was no better than pretend (placebo) surgery.[6] Arthroscopic surgery for simple osteoarthritis of the knees now has been eliminated, leading to both reduced cost and complications for patients.

Commonplace treatments like traction and prolonged bed rest for persistent low back pain, and antibiotics for the common cold, are also now avoided because they have been proved significantly less beneficial, and more harmful, than alternatives. No different than the resistance to medical modifications of old, however, the transition to graded progressive exercise programs to alleviate nonspecific back pain, and fluids and rest to combat the common cold, has not been well received, especially by patients. Uninformed, misled, or just plain stubborn, they push to "let their backs rest" or demand "a pill to kill the cold." For today's general practitioners, reeducating patients is not an easy task.

Early History of Psychiatric Treatment

As with general medical care, psychiatry's advance toward outcome-changing treatment has had its share of well-intended, but unfortunate, missteps. For centuries, many educated men and women concurred that people exhibiting abnormal behavior must be adversely affected during certain phases of the moon. The moon theory of madness spawned the terms *lunacy, lunatics,* and *loony bin* from the Latin word *lunar,* meaning "moon." Others, not buying into the moon theory, opined that sufferers of mental malfunction were being punished by God for their sins or, even worse, had been kidnapped by the devil. Assuming bodies without souls could feel no pain or cold or hunger, advocates of the possession theory worried themselves little about how to maintain the insane. Short of prayer, exorcism, incantation, or merciful death, no remedy was attempted beyond protecting the afflicted from self-harm or harm to others.

By the eighteenth century, more creative, though maybe not kinder, treatments developed. Benjamin Rush, the first U.S. general medical physician turned alienist invented the tranquilizing chair (Figure 2.2), which was quite effective in calming manic patients, but they could be confined to the chair for weeks at a time. Collapsing bridges that plunged patients into ice-cold water were used to shock them into sanity

Figure 2.2 Tranquilizing chair.
Before effective treatments for mental illness became available, Benjamin Rush, one of the first alienists in the United States, used the tranquilizing chair to control manic and psychotic behavior, sometimes for weeks.

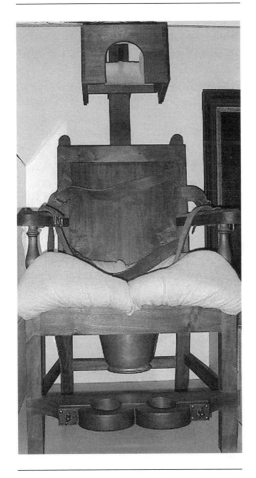

Source: Photo courtesy of Dr. Anthony Walsh, Chair, Department of Psychology, Salve Regina University, Newport, Rhode Island.

or to cool the overly warm humors of their minds. The Utica crib, (picture a baby bed with a locked lid), helped agitated patients rest. Tonics and potions, such as the Victorian-age narcotic laudanum, were given regularly to subdue hysteria.

Between 1930 and 1950, more sophisticated treatment attempts were introduced, like hydrotherapy (ice-water baths for three or more hours at a time), insulin shock therapy that rendered the patient unconscious due to lack of blood sugar, and frontal lobotomy. Although these early treatments have been replaced with treatments of greater efficacy and less risk to patients with similar problems, they were all associated with some clinical improvement. They were used to help patients with otherwise intractable behaviors, emotions, or sensory experiences. The alternative was a life sentence at the asylum and/or premature death for lack of any kind of care.

Though the bulk of these early efforts to address and alleviate behavioral health disorders have been abandoned, each trial improved our understanding of the underpinnings of mental disorders (psychopathology). As you will learn in later chapters, they were all, to one degree or another, trailblazers for the next generation of biological treatment in mentally ill patients and those with substance abuse problems.

Approaching mental illness and chemical dependence from a different angle, psychiatrists and clinical psychologists expanded their practice to include psychotherapeutic treatment for patients with less severe emotional conditions. Commonly known as *talk therapy,* the treatment was a twentieth-century blockbuster and a notable part of Western culture from its highest to lowest expression.

The young, ambitious neurologist Sigmund Freud eagerly joined the fascinating field of psychiatry upon which he left an indelible thumbprint by fathering insight-oriented psychotherapy, a term nearly synonymous with psychodynamic or psychoanalytic psychotherapy. He based his theory on the healing power of words, convinced that uncovering early traumatic life events would lead to insight. Insight would, in turn, relieve subconscious anxieties and reverse ineffective or disturbing coping mechanisms. Considering the truly insane, such as those with psychosis, mania, catatonia, and so forth, beyond hope, Freud limited his so-called talking cure to well-educated neurotic patients, whose mental conditions caused distress but did not interfere with rational thought or the ability to function.

Although Freud was the first, the number of theories about psychological etiologies for abnormal behaviors ultimately exploded, and tight cliquish psychotherapeutic camps formed. Though bickering among themselves, even today, about which early-life experiences were most important in the development of behavioral pathology and how to uncover them, most camps of talk therapists stood united in their opposition to biological therapies. They contended that the biological approach was impersonal, reductionistic, and neglected real issues in patients' lives that were core to symptom resolution. This rift between biological and psychotherapeutic proponents persists. More on this later.

MEDICAL PRACTITIONERS ASSUME TREATMENT RESPONSIBILITY FOR PHYSICAL ILLNESSES WITH PSYCHIATRIC MANIFESTATIONS

Medical records on disorders that led to admission to asylums in the mid-1800s (Table 2.1) indicate that about 10 percent to 15 percent of admitted patients had epilepsy, recognizable by limb and body shaking, emotional outbursts, and various fits and seizures. About 5 percent to 10 percent had general paresis, better known today as neurosyphilis, which in late stages (tertiary) causes marked

Table 2.1
Forms of Lunacy Circa 1850

Diagnosis in 1850	Approximate Present-day Equivalent
Mania	Mania
	Schizophrenia
Dementia	Dementia
Melancholia	Major depressive disorder
Monomania	Delusional (paranoid) disorder
Moral insanity	Alcohol and drug abuse
Prostitution	
Hysteria	
Idiocy/imbecility	Mental retardation
General paresis	Neurosyphilis
Epilepsy	Epilepsy

Note: Patients with epilepsy and neurosyphilis, treated in the mid-nineteenth century in asylums, are now entirely under the care of nonpsychiatrist physicians. Many other physical illnesses with behavioral manifestations also have switched from mental health to medical care as effective treatments have emerged.

and progressive nerve and mental degeneration secondary to brain deterioration. Motor incoordination, speech impairment, convulsions, mania, depression, paranoia, violent behavior, suicide, delusions, loss of memory, disorientation, and apathy are, alone or in combination, some of the ravages seen in patients with late untreated syphilis.

Tragically for many—because the symptoms for both epilepsy and neurosyphilis mirrored the symptoms of other mental disorders—lunacy, sin, or possession were invoked as causes, and the patients were usually incarcerated without treatment. With the introduction of the electroencephalogram (EEG), the bleak future of patients with epilepsy diagnosed as mentally ill brightened dramatically. In the early 1900s, a physical cause for epileptic fits could be documented. Further, a connection between patients with general paresis and the sexually transmitted disease syphilis was established.

Merging with the advances in testing capabilities, the availability of effective drug therapy for epilepsy and syphilis helped thin out the asylum population. A partial response to bromide in the late 1800s and slightly better outcomes with phenobarbital (Luminal), introduced in 1912, prompted a movement in which patients experiencing seizures would be transferred from asylums to specialty centers for epileptics. Driven more by the false worry that other mental patients could contract epilepsy by touching a patient during a seizure than by recognition that epilepsy is distinct from other mental conditions, the transition from asylum to a medical setting, nonetheless, was pivotal in the evolution of treatment for epileptic patients.

Though having epilepsy, like mental illness, still carries a stigma, its treatment has traveled a long way from the confines of a straightjacket.

Similar changes also occurred in the treatment for syphilis early in the twentieth century. Arsenic preparations and malaria-induced fevers for syphilis reduced admissions for lunacy related to neurosyphilis. Treatment of this venereal infection during its early phases did not occur with great regularity until late in World War II, however, when penicillin (discovered in 1928) became widely available. Penicillin was much less toxic than arsenic and did not subject a patient receiving fever therapy to a malaria infection that, in turn, necessitated treatment to prevent its complications.

Although epilepsy and syphilis were perhaps the most common medical illnesses seen in the behavioral health setting in the last half of the nineteenth century and early twentieth century, other common physical illnesses also were treated as mental disorders. Porphyria, encephalitis, brain tumors, rheumatic fever, Parkinson's disease, and Cushing's disease are but a few of the diseases that were treated in asylums. A couple of examples illustrate this situation nicely.

Advanced hyperthyroidism manifests symptoms difficult to distinguish from acute manic attacks. During periods of sharply elevated levels of thyroid hormone production, known as thyroid storms, heart rates soar, eyes bulge, body temperatures rise, hair thins, and skin flushes. The patient experiences emotional excitement and insomnia. Prior to the diagnostic and treatment era (circa 1875), many people exhibiting these symptoms were housed in asylums and often died of so-called manic exhaustion. Severe manic patients with bipolar illness in the era before electroconvulsive therapy, lithium, and antipsychotic agents regularly suffered the same fate.

Another good example of an illness, which has passed from psychiatry to internal medicine, is porphyria, the inherited enzyme deficiency that struck King George III in 1765. Had his doctors known then that psychiatric manifestations (agitation, irritability, psychosis, and incoherency) of the illness could have been prevented or, at least, attenuated early and easily with a change of diet, the poor king would not have endured the horrors of attempted cures. Quite possibly, on the right diet, he also might have avoided being immortalized as the king who "lost America" in the American Revolution.

Gradually over the years, evidence of, and in many cases treatment for, underlying physical diseases as causative or aggravating factors for the development of psychiatric symptoms motivated a shift of patients from psychiatrists to general medical professionals. Today, for most established medical illnesses with behavioral manifestations, early identification of the physical disorder and effective treatment now obviates the occurrence of mental health symptoms. Focus on early and effective treatment of the general medical condition is usually sufficient.

In today's world of medicine, porphyria and hyperthyroidism are eminently treatable; however, we find numerous bonified physical diseases with psychiatric manifestations that have no known medical treatment. Regrettably, many of these are also primarily treated in the non–mental health sector. Notable in this category, is Huntington's disease, an inherited condition that leads to personality change, abnormal physical movements (known as chorea), and occasionally psychosis. If the behavioral elements of the disease are not treated in conjunction with the physical components, serious complications can develop.

One of my most dangerous patients had Huntington's disease. A well-meaning and knowledgeable neurologist was caring for him. Remanded to treatment in my medical psychiatry unit, Mark was in a progressive delusional state. Convinced that his neighbors were spying on him, he arrived on their front porch armed with a shotgun and a chef's knife. Beating on the door, he raged, "I'll stop your abuse once and for all!"

Luckily, because of Mark's prior demonstrations of aggression, the neighbors had locks in place and immediately summoned police assistance before a crime occurred. Had his neurologist been trained in the dangers of and treatment for the psychiatric manifestations of the illness, and/or chosen to address them, the threatening psychotic situation with the neighbors could have been averted.

PROGRESS IN BEHAVIORAL HEALTH TREATMENT

This book is not intended to be a compendium of the progression in the efficacy of treatment for psychiatric conditions; however, it is important for the reader to appreciate the advances that have been made in assisting people with behavioral, cognitive, emotional, and substance-related disturbances. Fewer than 75 years ago, patients with mental illness were incarcerated to protect society from their troubling behavior and suffered unabated mental anguish as a result of their illness. Impaired by obsessions or compulsions, hallucinations, misuse of alcohol, recurrent thoughts of suicide, and many other symptoms, barriers to happiness and productivity were often persistent and insurmountable. Hope was a pipe dream.

Today, because of the great strides taken to understand the conditions of the mind and their relationship to the body, there is not only hope but also predictable success for many, if not most. To be sure, advances for care of patients with psychiatric illness have not kept even pace with advances in general medicine. One contributing factor to the lag is the routine migration of patients from psychiatric physicians to general medical physicians whenever a behavioral disturbance is related to a medical condition. A recent example of the shift is found for patients with dementia. With the availability of memory-enhancing medications, care of this population is rapidly moving from psychiatry to neurology and internal medicine. As a result of this and similar redistributions of patients, psychiatry finds itself continuously redefining the boundaries of its professional domain.

Another critical waylay has been psychiatry's difficulty in consistently defining patterns of behavior; that is, syndromes and ultimately diseases. Without epidemiological and/or treatment comparisons of homogenous samples (apples to apples), scientific investigation was not possible. The lack of sophisticated investigative tools to open the mind for study, as well as the scarcity of effective treatments for most psychiatric disorders before the second half of the twentieth century, also delayed psychiatric advancement.

Finally, and significantly, psychiatry's and psychology's love affair with psychodynamic explanations for abnormal emotions and behaviors (based on the assumption that abnormal response to early-life experiences causes psychiatric illness), together with myriad and varied offshoots of psychotherapy, has stifled progress and continues to do so. Within the culture of Oedipal conflicts and transference-countertransference, research and implementation of more valuable interventions for symptom reduction and/or reversal were soundly remitted to the back burner for years.

Because we will be moving toward the importance of not only integrating general medical and behavioral health care but also the coordination of biological and psychological interventions for mental and substance-use disorders, it is worth spending time providing a simplistic understanding of advances that have been made in psychological and biological treatments.

Psychological Interventions

In the 1890s, Freud hypothesized that human behavior is influenced by biological and psychological drives. Dismantling earlier beliefs that the full moon or sin led to mental dysfunction, Freud's writings ushered in the era of psychodynamic thinking. He emphasized sexuality and aggression as the prime motivators for aberrant behavior and concluded that psychiatric illness evolved from a person's early memories. Free association, hypnosis, and nondirective talk therapy were his tools. People with money and time to spare flocked (even today) to analysts' couches to recover memories of early-life experiences. Insight about the influence that early-life experiences had on behavior allegedly would then lead to correction of a maladaptive approach to life.

Psychoanalysis captured the imagination of some of the most brilliant psychiatric minds, many of whom postulated their own rendition of varying innate drives that led to mental illness. Carl Jung's individuation and collective consciousness, Alfred Adler's inferiority theory, and Melanie Klein's focus on human relationships all flowered and survive today.

Unfortunately, as with many treatments tried throughout medical history, like bone marrow transplantation and bloodletting, psychoanalytic psychotherapy has not lived up to expectations. If it were a medication, the Food and Drug Administration (FDA) would consider it experimental. To date, it has not demonstrated efficacy (does what it claims to do) or effectiveness (works consistently in clinical situations), both FDA requisites. It also has attendant dangers in terms of inaccurate accusations of early abuse by uncovering false memories, unpredictable and/or poor outcomes while neglecting alternative effective treatments, and the development of pathological dependency relationships between the patient and therapist.

Intuitively and experientially, we all know that life experiences, early and late, do influence a person's reaction to life circumstances. Studies have shown, however, that few predict the development of psychiatric illness. Library shelves groan with the weight of books written about very successful, well-adjusted people who lived through horrendous childhoods without the benefit of psychotherapy, whereas other accounts tell of individuals with golden childhoods who suffer with obsessive-compulsive disorder or panic attacks.

During my years as a practicing psychiatrist, I have treated scores of eating-disorder patients. Some of these individuals had received insight-oriented psychotherapy for years. Many revealed significant early-life traumas through this experience, whereas others could recollect none. Although they had gained tremendous insight into supposed traumatic childhood experiences in sessions with their long-term therapists, they came under my care because they were near death from malnutrition. The limited comparative studies of this form of psychotherapy published in behavioral health literature fail to support that insight-oriented therapy is better than no therapy at all.

Though a diversion from effective psychiatric care, just as laudanum and lobotomy, insight-oriented therapies do represent a step forward in that the patient, as a person, is considered as important as the illness in the reparative process. Undeniably, psychological and social aspects of human behavior are vital components of healing in health care, including but not limited to psychiatry. Long-term (measured in years) psychodynamic therapy, what I call *there-and-then therapy,* focuses on relationships, early-life experiences, social influences on behavior, and the interaction between clinician and patient. For this reason, the methodology has a modicum of merit, but only to the extent that it demonstrates predictable improvement and is usable for recognized psychiatric illness in terms of therapist time and resources available to support its use.

There-and-then therapies utilize an unstructured therapeutic environment wherein improvement can occur only if and when a patient gains insight into the relationship of the past to current emotional and behavioral difficulties. Without requiring the patient to take active steps toward resolution of the offending target behaviors and emotions, this type of therapy can go on for years with no guarantee of improvement. The hit-or-miss aspect of psychodynamic psychotherapy, of which formal psychoanalysis is one form, with its inherent roadblocks to usability and lack of efficacy, will predictably become obsolete, just as occurred with tranquilizing chairs and Utica cribs.

Their inclusion in the anthology of mental health advances, however, is advantageous. Drawing from improved understanding of human behavior, in part derived from insight-based therapies, *here-and-now therapies* are springing from the ashes. In here-and-now therapy, the distant past etiology of problems is less important than active involvement in techniques designed to help patients improve their own problematic behaviors. During the past twenty years, a number of evidenced-based here-and-now talk therapies, such as cognitive behavioral therapy (CBT), interpersonal psychotherapy (IPT), problem-solving therapy (PST), and dialectical behavior therapy (DBT), have gathered evidence of efficacy and momentum among psychotherapists and are gradually replacing there-and-then therapies.

Virtually all here-and-now therapies draw on so-called dynamic underpinnings; that is, maladaptive behaviors originating from learned experiences (Table 2.2). They emphasize and focus on the future, however, rather than the past. Relying on the principle that patients must learn new adaptive behaviors, CBT, IPT, PST, and

Table 2.2
Psychotherapy

Types (simplistic)

1. *Support and crisis intervention*
     • Listening and caring with availability and support through time of stress
     • Can be provided by any caring, concerned person either professional (e.g., doctor or nurse) or nonprofessional (e.g., family or friend)
     • Decreases suffering but does not predictably change outcome
     • In many ways synonymous with counseling

2. *There-and-then formal therapies*
     • Traditional yet still experimental because studies do not support efficacy
     • Common names for it:
             Psychoanalysis
             Insight-oriented therapy
             Long-term psychodynamic therapy

3. *Here-and-now formal therapies*
     • Proved efficacious in selected conditions
     • Examples:
             Cognitive behavioral therapy (CBT)
             Interpersonal psychotherapy (IPT)
             Problem-solving therapy (PST)
             Dialectical behavior therapy (DBT)

Key components for predictable outcome change

1. Positive relationship between patient (client) and clinician
2. A condition that can be expected to respond to therapy (e.g., anxiety or depression, but not schizophrenia)
3. Shared patient and clinician focus on time-sensitive therapeutic goals
4. Therapist adherence to critical manual-driven intervention components (here-and-now therapies) adapted to patient
5. Active involvement of the patient in learning and using therapeutic practices
6. An adequate number of sessions based on illness and intervention (usually 8 to 20 but can be longer for DBT in so-called out-of-control patients with borderline personality disorder)
7. An end point for therapy

Note: Not all psychotherapies are backed by evidence to support their effectiveness. Patients wishing to start or who are already receiving psychotherapy should review this simplistic breakdown of types of therapy and key outcome-related components to make sure that they have the greatest chance of improvement.

DBT all start with setting goals for therapy by establishing how the patient wishes to think, act, and feel in the future. Then, by learning techniques to accomplish those goals, the patient systematically implements new approaches using homework assignments during a prescribed period of time. Good therapists work with their patients toward resolution of symptoms, not just improvement. When this is not possible, then maximizing adaptation given unchangeable impairment becomes the goal. The intent is always on patients reclaiming control of their lives through the techniques they learn, followed by a timely closure of the therapeutic relationship.

For instance, CBT uses techniques that challenge cognitive distortions leading to depression or anxiety. It teaches patients strategies to counter these distorted thoughts and expects them to try out new approaches (behaviors) in real-life situations over 8 to 16 weekly therapy sessions. Using this action-based methodology has proved equally effective to antidepressant medications in those with mild to moderate depression. Furthermore, CBT has been shown to augment outcomes in those who have only a partial response to medication. IPT uses a participatory goal-oriented approach centered on relationships, and PST simplistically explores and tries out alternative behaviors to those considered as contributors to the current problem.

DBT, developed for people with a severe and debilitating problem in forming stable personal relationships, self-injurious impulsive actions, and a chaotic and unpredictable lifestyle (borderline personality disorder), takes more time. It, too, however, establishes goals, requires performance of homework assignments, uses milestones to monitor and document progress, and has an end point.

Those receiving any of the forms of here-and-now therapy may continue less frequent so-called reinforcement sessions after the completion of the formal phase of treatment, just as it is necessary to reinforce and support adherence in patients with difficult-to-treat hypertension, asthma, and/or diabetes. The objective of CBT, DBT, and so forth is for patients to learn therapeutic techniques sufficiently well that they can automatically reactivate learned strategies to counter future episodes without the need for therapist-based assistance. Here-and-now therapies are a major advance in the psychological approach to a number of selected, but by no means all, psychiatric difficulties.

Perhaps the major problem with here-and-now psychotherapies is that many therapists in today's therapeutic environment do not use them as they are intended. Therapists need to apply the critical components of the intervention for change to happen. Although therapists may say that they are employing CBT, IPT, PST, or DBT, many consider the core features of these concretely directed treatments too confining. Reverting to a more seductive dynamic approach with focus on uncovering detrimental early-life experiences and pursuing ill-defined goals is not uncommon.

Some therapists also lack adequate training. In fact, inconsistently standardized training among psychologists, social workers, and other therapists from state to state (U.S.) and country to country is currently a major problem when one wishes to assure that referral for psychological intervention has a likelihood of behavior change. Even MD- and PhD-level professionals may not have the clinical background and training necessary to provide outcome-changing here-and-now therapy. They find here-and-now therapies too complicated to administer or have no systematic experience in using them.

When this happens, therapists do the best they can, mostly by providing support and crisis intervention (see Table 2.2). They listen to patients describe current problematic life situations, such as marital difficulties, job loss, or loneliness. A discussion about coping skills may follow, but with no defined goals related to underlying difficulties, such as depression, anxiety, eating disorder, and so forth. All too often, nonconformance to core principles of here-and-now therapies predicts delayed response or nonresponse.

Another well-recognized drawback to all talk therapies, and particularly here-and-now therapies, is that the process demands patient involvement. The homework assignments designed to control or improve patient-specific activities, such as suicidal gestures, binge drinking, or sabotaging personal relationships, are crucial to success. Even with the most ideal doctor-patient relationships in which the patients fully understand the important role they play in the therapeutic process, adherence to homework assignments is not an insignificant hurdle to overcome. Any general practitioner who recommends smoking cessation or weight reduction in the general medical clinic will attest to this. All psychotherapies are active processes and require motivation, sufficient intelligence, and participation in order to succeed. There is no pixie dust.

Patients have numerous reasons for nonadherence. Some patients do not believe learning new behaviors, as occurs in the psychotherapeutic process, is worth the effort or even possible. In these cases, patients do not show up for appointments or will not do the work needed outside of therapy sessions to improve symptoms and change outcome. Other patients may be too ill to become actively involved. For instance, patients with psychosis may be too impaired to communicate coherently. Patients suffering with anhedonia, a symptom of depression that squelches all interest in doing things, will have no inclination to follow through.

The good news is that for the selected common behavioral disorders, such as mild to moderate depression and anxiety, talk-therapy approaches can change long-term outcomes either alone or in combination with medication. Patients willing to put forth the effort, presuming they can find a therapist who gives one of the manualized here-and-now therapies, can be treated in 8 to 20 weekly sessions, a substantial reduction in time and cost when compared to the years that there-and-then therapy requires.

Furthermore, if patients work hard in learning the therapy techniques, it is possible that they can prevent and/or attenuate future difficulties. Importantly, the addition of here-and-now psychotherapy to medication or medication to here-and-now psychotherapy appears to lead to greater benefit than either intervention alone in partial responders or in those with treatment resistance.

Biological Interventions

Effective treatment in biological psychiatry was ushered in by the shock therapies. Physicians used insulin shock around 1930, Metrazol shortly thereafter, and eventually the more controllable electroconvulsive therapy (ECT). Thanks to misleading popular movies like *Shock Corridor, One Flew Over the Cuckoo's Nest,* and *Frances,* a stench of barbarism trails ECT but does not diminish its lifesaving capabilities. Induction of seizures by applying low-dose electric shock over the temples was the first consistent and usable advance in treatment for seriously ill patients with disabling psychiatric symptoms, particularly mania, psychotic depression, and catatonia.

Before the availability of ECT, these disorders led to malnutrition and other illness in individuals who could not take care of themselves or necessitated a lifetime in mental hospitals with years of suffering. In the most severe cases, early death from manic exhaustion or suicide ensued. Still used today is a refined modification of ECT in which physical manifestations of seizure are largely blocked by a medication (neuromuscular blocker), and the administration of the electrical impulse is more precisely controlled and patient-friendly.

Lithium, the first medication for manic-depressive (bipolar) illness circa 1940, and chlorpromazine (commonly known as Largactil or Thorazine), the first approved antipsychotic agent circa 1950, followed ECT as effective treatments for seriously psychotic patients. Imipramine, a synthesized derivative of medications like chlorpromazine, along with iproniazid, an antitubercular agent, were medications introduced to treat depression shortly thereafter.

Refinements in our understanding of psychiatric diagnosis paralleled improvements in the use of these biological therapies, making it possible to better delineate behavioral syndromes. Using clearly defined and reproducible (criteria-based) behavioral syndrome descriptions, the historical progression and/or intermittent appearance of symptoms, evidence for a positive family history of similar illness, and response to treatment, future psychiatric difficulties could be projected. Psychiatrists treating patients with severe mental illness were finally comparable to their physical health colleagues. They now had scientifically based studies that demonstrated diagnostic reliability and treatments that predictably improved outcomes. Further, they could now test new and promising interventions using reproducible methodologies.

Since the mid-twentieth century, psychiatric conditions and subcategories of conditions have been defined and redefined in much the same way that general medicine updates information about its disorders. For example, schizophrenia, affective disorder, chemical dependence, dementia, and eating disorders all have gone through numerous revisions about how each illness is identified and who fits into the clinical syndrome in revisions of the American Psychiatric Association's *Diagnostic and Statistical Manual of Mental Disorders (DSM)*.

The manual is now in its fourth edition *(DSM-IV)*, almost unrecognizable when compared to the first. These editions are updated when new information warrants. The latest text-revised version is called *DSM-IV-TR*.[7] Advances in categorization of mental illness for the first time put the diagnosis and treatment of psychiatric illness on even scientific footing with the rest of medicine.

With the right medication or combination of medications, the majority of schizophrenic and paranoid patients who are troubled with hallucinations, delusions, and other psychotic manifestations now can depend on at least symptom reduction, if not symptom elimination. Furthermore, earlier medications that transformed patients into zombies have been replaced with equally or more effective medications that have less serious appearance-altering side effects.

Medications with proved effectiveness also are available now for depression, anxiety disorders, and mania. Even in patients with traditional treatment-resistant disorders, such as dementia and chemical dependence, we are finding medications that contribute to improved outcomes. For instance, studies using cholinesterase and N-methyl-D-aspartate (NMDA) receptor antagonists indicate that progression of memory impairment can be retarded and in some cases reversed (at least for a short time).[8]

Methadone reverses medical and social morbidity associated with chronic narcotic abuse. Buprenorphine is shown to decrease future narcotic abuse potential.[9] The addition of naltrexone or acamprosate to traditional alcohol dependence treatment in individuals at high risk for future abuse decreases return to heavy drinking by nearly a third when compared to those who do not receive it.[10] With medications, such as bupropion and nortriptyline, we also are finding that we can improve risk behaviors not associated with mental illness, such as smoking. Medications used for mental illness and substance-use disorders have come a long way since their introduction in the 1940s and 1950s.

Medications and ECT form the mainstay of biological therapies and are used effectively to reverse symptoms of psychosis, depression, anxiety, mania, and other mental disturbances that cause suffering and impair function. Other biological interventions are in the wings. We now use phototherapy (full-spectrum lights) for seasonal affective disorder. Vagus-nerve, transcranial-magnetic, and, most recently, deep-brain stimulation of the subgenual cingulate region show promise in treating depression and, perhaps, other psychiatric conditions. Transcranial magnet-induced seizures also offer promise as a low-side-effect alternative to electrically induced seizures for severe depression.

Since the mid-1990s, surgical interventions for intractable obsessive-compulsive and bipolar disorder have shown some benefit in a portion of the small number of patients who receives them. Though little in the way of side effects or surgical complications have been reported, cutting nerve connections in the brain, such as with stereotactic cingulotomy and other surgical approaches like it, remains an intervention that requires further study. In the next decade, some of the most promising treatments for all health care disciplines will likely, however, be in the area of gene-substitution therapy.

Synthesis of Psychological and Biological Interventions

In his *Foundation* trilogy, Isaac Asimov introduced psychohistorian Hari Seldon, who described a rarely occurring life-/worldview-changing event, known as the Seldon Crisis. With the advances that have transpired in the identification and treatment of psychiatric disorders, behavioral health clinicians (psychotherapists, those specializing in biological interventions, or those doing both), their physical health physician colleagues, and the patients they serve are on the cusp of their own Seldon Crisis. Unfortunately, what has not occurred in the current behavioral health environment is widespread recognition of the value that the systematic application of combined outcome-changing biological/psychotherapeutic (biopsychosocial) approaches in the physical health and psychiatric setting bring to those suffering from mental and/or substance-use disorders.

A significant percentage of the 35,000 psychiatrists and 120,000 psychologists in the United States, many with political connections and power, remain enamored with non-evidence-based psychotherapeutic explanations for, and approaches to, abnormal emotions, cognitions, and behaviors. The reductionistic method, whereby every patient's problem now can be categorized using a diagnostic label, is intolerable to many of these practitioners. As well, many have a palpable aversion to biological interventionists, who, in their opinion, "just drug clients up." (Therapists often use the word *client* for *patient*.)

Fixed on environment as the primary inciting factor for psychiatric illness, many of my colleagues, espousing psychotherapy over biological therapies, continue to insist that medications are poisonous and that ECT causes irreversible brain damage. They argue that biological psychiatrists consider problematic mental and substance-use disorders mere alterations in brain substrate yet dismiss the major role life experiences and circumstances play in symptom development and subsequent resolution. An oft-repeated mantra is that biological clinicians focus on the illness at the expense of the patient.

Within this hotbed of debate, frustrated by the paucity of psychotherapists with outcome-changing therapy skills in CBT, IBT, PST, and DBT, a growing number of biopsychosocially oriented psychiatrists are interested in addressing psychiatric illness with biological therapies in combination with psychotherapy. During limited medication management time slots, they try to provide the blend of therapies, but their effort is thwarted by the carved-out behavioral health reimbursement system, which will be explained in detail later. It confines these specialists to 15-minute impersonal outpatient visits or pays substantially less if longer time intervals are used. The message is clear: "Adjust the medication and don't talk with the patient, stupid."

Unfortunately, the ongoing nature-versus-nurture debate deepens the schism within the behavioral health community, fueling competition between the biological camp and psychological camp for funding, patients, and recognition. As well, dissonance within the behavioral health field, including the arguments from a few leftovers from the possessed-by-the-devil theory, does not shine a reassuring light to the physical health community. The schism undermines progress in integrating medical and behavioral health services.

Between 1988 and 1998, the percentage of the health care dollar devoted to behavioral health care plummeted from more than 6 percent to 3 percent of the total health care dollar spent. In some markets today, it is as low as 2 percent. No surprise! The internal friction of bickering behavioral health specialists (Table 2.3) has worked against itself, creating an ideal environment for those who do not believe that mental or substance-use disorders are treatable conditions and who wish to minimize support for this area of medical practice. Divide and Conquer!

Substantial and long-recognized evidence purports a profound relationship between behavioral difficulties and physical illness, a connection that ultimately affects the health of the whole person. With a medical headline of such magnitude and consequence, one would logically anticipate a brisk dialogue of ideas to ignite between mental health providers and physical health practitioners, but this has not been the case. For thirty years, organized general medicine has chosen to

Table 2.3
Behavioral Health Personnel

Psychiatrists—medical doctors (MD or DO) specializing in mental and substance-use disorders

Knowledge base
Physiological and psychological basis for behavioral manifestations of physical illness and medications; major and minor behavioral, emotional, and cognitive disturbances; research
Interventions
Psychotherapy, medications for mental and substance-use disorders, light therapy, electroconvulsive therapy, vagal stimulation, other
Subspecialties
Child and adolescent, substance-use disorders, geriatrics, psychosomatic medicine, forensic, or with dual training in family practice, pediatrics, internal medicine, neurology

Psychologists—nonmedically trained specialists in mental and substance-use disorders

Knowledge base
Psychological aspects of mental and substance-use disorders; neurocognitive and neuropsychological testing; psychological, organizational, and developmental assessments; research

Educational levels
Doctoral (PhD, EdD, PsyD), master's or bachelor's (special license or supervision for clinical practice)

Interventions
Psychotherapy, biofeedback, hypnosis, behavior change techniques

Subspecialties
Clinical (health, neuropsychology, geropsychology, counseling), school, industrial-organizational, developmental, social, research

Psychiatric nurses—medically trained nurses specializing in mental and substance-use disorders

Knowledge base
Medical and psychological problem resolution for psychiatric disturbances whether related to medical or psychiatric disease; (APN—advanced training in physiology, psychology, and psycho-pharmacology of mental illness and substance-use disorders)
Educational levels
Advanced practice nurses (APN), clinical nurse specialists (CNS), registered nurses (RN)

Interventions
Variable up to level of APN that can have prescribing and independent decision-making privileges

Subspecialties
Adult, child and adolescent, family, public health

Social workers—nonmedically trained specialists (MSW, other) who assist clients through socially difficult situations
Knowledge base
Social and environmental problems and system issues that affect a person's life

Interventions
Assisting with supportive counseling and crisis intervention, discharge planning, community and health care resource utilization; some also obtain psychotherapy skills
Subspecialties
Family and school, medical and public health, mental and substance-use disorders

Other behavioral health personnel—substance-use disorder counselor, marriage and family therapist, counselor, practical nurse, etc.

Note: Behavioral health practitioners have diverse training and expertise, as summarized here, thus they are not interchangeable. Predictable improvement of mental health and substance-use disorders requires that care be delivered by clinicians who have the necessary skill sets to effect change.

distance itself from psychiatric care. And why not? If behavioral health specialists can not agree on a cause or treatment for mental disturbances, what benefit would be gained from the input of the physical health community whose expertise lies outside the purview of mental and substance-use disorders?

In spite of the warring camps pushing their own brands of diagnosis and treatment, hope remains. Integration is possible and currently lies in a synthesis of advances in both psychological and biological treatments coordinated with general medical care. Because behavioral health care's diagnostic capabilities and treatments are at long last on par with other medical disciplines, the time is ripe to integrate the medical system. Another compelling reason to escalate the campaign toward integration is that the bulk of reliable research now confirms that untreated psychiatric illness in medical patients perpetuates physical health treatment resistance, complexity, and complications.

To drive this point home, recall Harry from Chapter 1. What would have happened if Harry had been exposed to brief intervention for alcohol dependence[11] (Table 2.4) early in the course of his drinking by his primary care physician? One might expect that his drinking, as suggested by published reports, would have subsided and the course of his liver failure to, at least, have been impeded. If brief intervention itself did not work, he would have been more likely to have been admitted into a formal substance-use disorder treatment program. Naltrexone and/or acamprosate also could have been prescribed to augment Harry's efforts to curb the urge to drink, decreasing his likely return to excessive drinking by a third. In today's separate health system paradigm, none of these alternatives were made available to Harry.

Table 2.4
Brief Intervention for Alcohol Dependence

Professional encounters
 Two primary care physician visits one month apart
 Two nurse calls two weeks after each physician visit

Intervention
 Workbook on health behaviors
 Review prevalence of problem drinking
 List adverse effects of alcohol
 Work sheet on drinking cues
 Prescription pad, drinking agreement
 Drinking diary cards

Outcome
 Less alcohol intake and abuse
 Greater entry into alcoholism treatment programs, if needed

Note: Brief intervention for alcohol abuse and dependence, the components of which have been summarized here, when provided by general practitioners and their staff has been shown to substantially reduce alcohol intake, progression to alcohol-related complications, and lower health care costs. Even when excessive alcohol intake remains a problem, there is a greater likelihood of entry into formal substance-use disorder treatment programs by graduates of brief intervention programs.

In Harry's predicament, perhaps the more important question to ask is "Why was Harry even offered the option of excluding substance-use disorder treatment from his health plan policy?" This is a common occurrence when independent business practices are used to manage behavioral health. Health coverage for heart disease and cancer are not options for exclusion to lower premium costs, yet substance abuse is. In Chapter 3, we will explore the long arm of contradictions, fractures, and factions intrinsic in a segregated medical system.

The journey into the science of medicine has been long and fraught with obstacles and mistakes, debates and dissensions, but the most memorable have been the breakthroughs. In retrospect, it is remarkable how similar the science of the body is to the science of the mind. Treatment of both began in ignorance of illness. The human body was a puzzle to dissect and discover. On the medical side, we reflect on Hippocrates' four humors and respective treatments:

> Blood: warm and moist.
>
> Phlegm: cold and moist.
>
> Yellow bile: warm and dry.
>
> Black bile: cold and dry.

Medical treatment was based on inaccurate knowledge of anatomy, and use of nonsterile surgical tools was part of routine care. Bleeding and moxibustion were named among the hierarchy of medical marvels. On the psychiatry side, incantations, exorcisms, executions, chains and cells, ice water, and starvation played enormous roles in treatment. Both disciplines relied heavily on medicinals, electricity, magnets, and other imaginative and infamous tools to restore health.

Today it is possible to cure bacterial pneumonia, stave off wound infections, replace missing hormones and prevent the overproduction of others, cut out diseased organs and transplant new ones, avoid unwanted pregnancies, and correct protein and chemical deficiencies. And now we are on the cusp of gene sequencing that potentially can prevent or correct abnormalities before they even occur.

Specific to the field of mental health, major advances in technology allow better understanding, not just of the anatomy of the brain but of the relationship of brain function to behavior. As a result, identification and treatment of many of the most common psychiatric conditions are now as good, if not better, as those available for the physical illnesses with which they are associated.

The most important lesson learned during the tests and trials of health care, regardless whether the treatment is for physical illness, mental and/or substance-use disorders, or a combination of both, is the relationship between the patient and his or her doctor, nurse, and/or therapist. This relationship is tantamount for predicting improvement and ensuring quality care. With this in mind, all of medicine, including psychiatry, now embarks on a seemingly new science in which we assess readiness for change and use motivational interviewing to help patients adhere to beneficial treatments and encourage them to help themselves through the episode of illness.

Recalling techniques of simpler days, before the advent of test machines and scientifically effective treatments, Dr. John Abramson describes the true art of doctoring in his book *Overdosed America*. His patient suffering with osteoarthritis came to him with worsening symptoms in her left knee joint. Although the medical press pushed the use of fancy scientific technology and expensive medications, Dr. Abramson recognized that a better solution for his patient was to modify her exercise regime. Having established a strong doctor-patient relationship with her over the years, he knew she needed a physical release to control recurrent anxiety. To avoid putting her on antianxiety agents, he encouraged her to replace her daily walk with aquatic exercises. This simple, noninvasive, and inexpensive recommendation allowed his patient to remain active and fit while her knee pain improved.

Despite the significant interaction of medical and behavioral misfires, body and mind specialists rarely interact, and herein lies a critical fault of our current health care system. There remain those behavioral health specialists who guard the function/dysfunction of the mind as if it were gang turf and those physical health practitioners who consider anatomical or physiological illnesses exclusively their domain. The time has come to gather the puzzle pieces and work as a team. Evidence mounts daily that the disconnect of body and mind in treating illness peppers the population with poor clinical outcomes and excessive health care costs. In the next chapter, we will take a closer look at the health system to see how it supports or creates barriers for patients in distress.

Chapter 3

HEALTH CARE MANAGEMENT

I know that you believe you understand what you think I said, but I'm
not sure you realize that what you heard is not what I meant.[1]
—Robert McCloskey

The young doctor tipped his hat and accepted the farmer's plumpest hen in payment
for his midnight ride to bring down a fever. In the early 1950s, pregnancy cost
the proud parents $150 start to finish. Dr. Roy, the GP down the street, treated
everything from mumps to broken bones, acne to blue moods, and never forgot
a birthday. But, like "Hi-Ho Silver" and candy cigarettes, those days are gone.
Forever. So are city-states and hunter-gatherers. Imagination and innovation
have moved mankind from caves into the age of technology. Technology has
opened the floodgate of scientific achievement.

Extraordinary advances in medicine have raised the U.S. life expectancy to
an all-time high—77.6 years—and deaths from heart disease, cancer, and stroke
continue to drop.[2] The discovery of gene imbalances has given hope to patients
with cystic fibrosis and soon could do the same for those with chronic alcoholism,
schizophrenia, and bipolar illness. Evidence-based therapies promise productive
lives for people suffering from once debilitating, if not deadly, mental health and
substance-use disorders.

The list of health milestones is impressive, but has not come without a price.
The vast quantity of intricate specifics about human anatomy, including the elabo-
rate wiring of the mind, is too much for one person to learn in medical school.
Specialization answered the dilemma. Though specialized medicine offers great
advantage in longer, healthier lives, the simplicity of health care disappeared and
costs have soared.

Contributing to skyrocketing health care costs is the expanding population; high-tech specialists, tests, and procedures; medications; and medical lawsuits, all leading to budget-busting medical cost inflation compared to spending for the U.S. gross domestic product.[3] In addition, the sheer magnitude of cost-shifting to settle the bill for those who use large amounts of high-dollar services and do not pay for them severely inflates doctor, hospital, and clinic fees. In response, health administrators in the 1980s replaced fee-for-service, or indemnity insurance, with a system that managed care. In the pure form of the managed care model, health plans are paid a fixed per-member-per-month (PMPM) fee by purchasers to manage all patient health expenses.

The impetus behind managed care was to identify and eliminate:

- Money squandered on doctors and hospitals that milked the system by performing unnecessary and expensive procedures.
- Drug and medical equipment companies that charged usurious prices.
- Patients who used excessive and expensive services because insurance companies and government agencies would "pick up the tab."

The managed care revolution was initially applauded by paying patients. It promised continuity of care, prevention, and early intervention at affordable health premiums. Heralded by a shift in decision-making power from clinicians to health plans, however, the cost-cutting strategies failed to cut costs in the long run and now provide a far lower quality product than prophesized.

Finally, in the previous chapter, we examined the limited interaction between the practitioners of behavioral and physical health care, even though the overlap of illnesses and their complications is pronounced. Accumulating studies now conclusively support the appropriateness of integration (to be discussed later), yet the division remains. A substantial contribution to this continued partition can be explained by an additional and convoluted component of managed care: an exclusionary managed behavioral health care system, which operates parallel to but independent from the physical health system. As will be reviewed, this artificial separation perpetuates *dis-integration* and the stigma of behavioral health in the physical health world with little hope of future substantive change.

In a maze of complexity, the stakeholders that create the infrastructure of virtually every health system worldwide (Figure 3.1)[4] serve as anchor points for understanding the challenges we face in the United States. The stakeholders include purchasers, fund distributors, providers, and patients.

- Purchasers buy health care access for constituents, employees, or themselves. They include government purchasing with tax dollars, employers purchasing with employee benefit deductions, organizations by way of fees charged to their members, and individuals paying out of pocket for health plan packages.

Figure 3.1 Health care infrastructure.
Purchasers, fund distributors, providers, and patients participate in a dynamic and interactive process, which affects the value brought to patients in health care systems throughout the world. Although it is what happens between doctors and their patients that directly influences disease and/or symptom resolution, the way that financial and administrative stakeholders support doctors in this effort influences the health of the populations served. Importantly, in most health systems worldwide, behavioral health is separated from the rest of medical care.

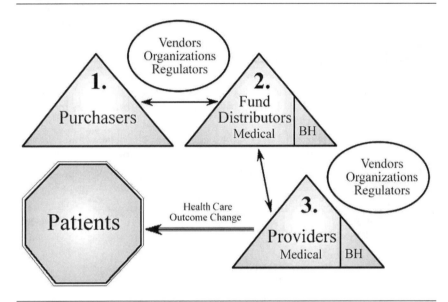

Source: Adapted from R. Kathol and D. Clarke, "Rethinking the Place of the Psyche in Health: Toward the Integration of Health Care Systems," *Australian and New Zealand Journal of Psychiatry* 39 (2005): 816–825.

- Fund distributors are health plans (once referred to as insurance companies) and government agencies, such as Medicare. The slender behavioral health (BH) divider in the figure denotes that the small amount of behavioral business is managed and paid for completely separately from general medical care. (Throughout the book the term *fund distributor* will be used interchangeably with the term *health plan*.)

- Providers include doctors, hospitals, clinics, therapists, nursing homes, rehabilitation centers, and any other professional, location, or organization that provides health services to patients. Again, care for mental health and substance-use disorders is largely dispensed independently from physical health care even though the same patient may be receiving treatment at the same time for both.

- Patients are enrollees of a government program, subscribers in a health plan, or the uninsured.

Simply put, purchasers buy coverage from fund distributors. Fund distributors pay providers, who treat patients. Uninsured patients receive necessary treatment as a requirement of law. The cost of care, when uninsured patients have no money, is shifted to those who pay in the form of increased premiums or higher taxes.

How the organization of this infrastructure works affects how patients receive treatment. In this chapter, we will explain the mechanics of one of the largest enterprises in the United States—health care—and how it defeats its own purpose.

HEALTH CARE INFRASTRUCTURE—THE BIG PICTURE

Although this book is written with an emphasis on health care in the United States, the infrastructure and the problems related to the separation of physical and behavioral health are as applicable to patients in Japan, Australia, and the Netherlands as they are to those in the United States. Each country has purchasers, fund distributors, providers, and patients. Each has a goal to promote a healthy population. And, curiously, virtually all consider treatment of mental health and substance-use disorders peripheral to the so-called real problems in the health care industry.

If, indeed, the goal is a healthy population, behavioral health is actually as important an area to debate in health care reform as pharmacy costs, provider reimbursement levels, and the administrative model used to support treatment in hospitals and clinics. No longer is it legitimate to lump evidence-based behavioral health care with acupuncture, naturopathy, and other forms of so-called alternative medicine health care approaches in restricting access and payment. If improved outcomes and reduced costs are desired, compelling evidence demands that people with psychiatric illness be treated in coordination with coexisting medical illness.

A crash course in the basic framework of medical care management is key to understanding the separate behavioral health system and its interaction with general medicine.

Purchasers (Employers, Government Programs, Individuals)

Purchasers buy access to health care services from fund distributors with specific goals in mind. For instance, when a branch of government accepts fiduciary responsibility, as occurs for individuals covered by Medicare or Medicaid (and most countries with nationalized health systems), staying within the appropriated annual budget is a priority. Employers, though also constrained by a budget, have a slightly different priority. Because time off work is money lost, they want their employees healthy and productive. Waiting lists and poor access to clinic appointments, hospitalization, tests, and procedures cut into employee productivity, and to this extent employers are more willing to spend extra health dollars for expediency and quality. Individuals, who buy their own insurance, either through an organization or directly from a fund distributor, want hassle-free quality care at a reasonable price.

Whether purchasers are agents of the Centers for Medicare and Medicaid Services (CMS), purchasing teams in companies such as IBM or the Dayton Corporation, or individuals representing their own interests, each must have a composite understanding of the health system in order to buy first-rate health care from their fund distributor. Purchasing health care coverage could be as simple as picking a plan and paying for it. But simple, it is not. Because fund distributors create products that come in all shapes and sizes and vary in price, coverage, and fee schedules, picking the right plan for a specific group or an individual is usually very complex.

Few purchasing negotiators have the training or sufficient information to know which plans fit within budget parameters and also translate into long-term health services that will lead to a healthy constituency. This problem is compounded by the fact that those who distribute funds tend to be the primary source when questions about what would be good arise—a bit like asking the fox how to guard the hen house. The task of fund distributors is to *manage* patient claims and pay providers. To do so, they establish solid business practices associated with a favorable expense-to-income ratio with profit their primary goal.

Health plan sales representatives promote products du jour by emphasizing short-term savings, such as lower pharmacy costs, larger provider discounts, and benefit restrictions. They neglect, however, to mention that standard by-products of cost shaving can be protracted illness, increased complications, higher readmission rates, and more expensive service use later. Of course, they fail to measure these by-products.

Purchasers who end up buying a less than satisfactory product can not necessarily blame the fund distributors. After all, purchasers of health care are fund distributor clients, and any worthwhile business will identify the needs of their clients and attempt to create a product that meets those demands within the guidelines of profit-taking. Today, most purchasers are fixated on cost with marching orders to decrease health care costs "this quarter," "by the end of the year," or "before the annual report comes out." Fund distributors design their products to accommodate. Unfortunately, short-term savings are usually at the expense of long-term savings generated by such things as improved employee productivity or enrollee readmission rates.

Individuals are also purchasers and include the self-employed, small business owners, students, early retirees, and part-time employees. Purchasers like the government and large corporations can negotiate health contracts with deep discounts because they represent large populations, but small groups and unaffiliated individuals have little negotiating leverage. Their rates are based on a limited risk pool and can be outrageous when individuals with serious or chronic illness buy the same product. Further, without human resource personnel or government agencies helping decipher confusing health plan verbiage, these do-it-yourselfers rarely understand what exactly they are buying.

After a while, they grow weary of trying to determine if their gynecologist, ophthalmologist, and psychiatrist are in the same provider network, if a higher deductible is worth a lower monthly premium, or if one company over another is more likely to hike rates. To avoid personal bankruptcy, in the event of illness or accident, they write a fat check every month to pay the premium, but even then there is no protection guarantee. According to a study of family bankruptcies filed in 2001, half were related to medical expenses, and three-quarters of those filing had health insurance before they lost their family savings.[5]

Because of their enormous drain on the health care bank, worthy of mention are potential purchasers: the uninsured. In the United States, where car insurance is mandatory, health coverage is not. Approximately 15 percent of the population go without it, and, contrary to popular thought, more than half of the estimated 46 million people who choose not to purchase insurance for themselves or their families are wage earners with incomes at least double the federal poverty level.[6]

The uninsured create a special challenge in the United States because by law anyone who needs urgent care must be given it. Because many of this group come to emergency rooms with preexisting conditions or do not access service early enough, they end up among those considered complex, high-cost patients. The expense of their treatment, in or out of an emergency room, is also often double that for insured patients because they do not benefit from health plan–generated network provider allowable discounts.

If they are without attachable assets (excluding their homes), then someone else has to pay for their services in order to keep hospitals, clinics, and providers from going out of business. In the form of higher premiums and inflated provider and testing charges, the people who have insurance pay the tab. The proverbial $15 box of Kleenex on the hospital bill is a perfect example of this type of cost shifting. As well, every taxpayer shoulders the burden through government subsidies and bailouts. An example is the tax-generated lump sums paid to hospitals that give care to a higher percentage of uninsured and underinsured in their region (disproportionate share funds).

Now enters the issue of the purchase of behavioral health coverage. Though at first glance it appears to be handled the same as the rest of medical coverage, nothing could be farther from the truth. Rates for coverage of mental health and substance-use disorders are usually negotiated in conjunction with physical health care, but there the connection ceases. Behavioral health coverage is dealt with as an appendage, offered as optional, and frequently (80%) purchased from an alternative company, such as United Behavioral Health, Magellan, ValueOptions, apart from the principle fund distributor, such as United Health Group, Blue Cross and Blue Shield of Virginia, Humana.

Purchasers at all levels typically view coverage for mental health and substance-use disorders differently than they do physical health care. Most, in fact, buy into the behavioral health myths drummed into their heads by fund distributor sales personnel. These myths suggest: (1) that the diagnosis and treatment of psychiatric illness occurs more often than it should; (2) that psychiatric illness is too sensitive for clinical notes to be shared with general medical clinicians also taking care of them and too complicated for them to treat it, thus special privacy measures for behavioral health information are paramount and practice locations are separated (more on this later); (3) that most behavioral disorders are untreatable; and (4) that concurrent psychiatric illness has little or no impact on physical health outcomes or cost. As a result, to ensure that unnecessary funds are not squandered treating illness that is overdiagnosed, incurable, and too personal to talk about, many pur-chasers are all too willing to buy into the additional myth that they are saving money by acquiring bare-bones mental health and substance-use disorder ser-vices. As we will see, a consistent decrease in behavioral health costs ultimately leads to overall higher total costs of care.

Fund Distributors (Health Plans and the Government)

With the advent of managed care, health plans look quite different than the fee-for-service insurance companies of yesteryear. Over the past thirty years, there has been a pronounced shift in payment formulas from protection to control. The management practices that fund distributors implement in the managed care environment are designed to prevent: (1) unethically high charges by providers, pharmaceutical companies, and medical device manufacturers and (2) wanton and indiscriminate use of excessive medical services by patients. To correct these transgressions, stringent cost-cutting features have amassed. Many of these sav-ings features are now familiar terms in our everyday health care lexicon. A short list of the most common includes:

- **Preferred provider networks:** providers agree to negotiated discounts for ser-vices delivered and become a part of a restricted provider network for insured patients. Higher prices (co-pays, coinsurance, and deductibles) are charged directly to members or enrollees when out-of-network providers are used, such as clinicians, hospitals, or clinics that have not agreed to negotiated discounts.

- **Fully insured plans:** insurance coverage in which the health plan makes the rules about benefits included in a plan and assumes financial risk for enrollee health service usage. One-third with commercial health insurance have this type of coverage.

- **Self-insured plans:** insurance coverage in which the purchaser, such as General Motors, the Carlson Company, the Department of Human Services, and so forth, makes the rules about benefits included in the plan and assumes financial risk for enrollee health service usage. Self-insured plans have greater flexibility under Employee Retirement Income Security Act (ERISA) laws about what they are required to cover; for example, substance-use disorder and mental health cover-age can be excluded. Two-thirds of the commercially insured are covered under these plans.

- **Utilization management** (often referred to by providers as the "just say no" approach to cost containment): fund distributors hire health professionals (usu-ally nurses) to review member service use to determine if a requested procedure or medical device is inappropriate or excessive (medically unnecessary as deter-mined by the fund distributor medical policy after review of pertinent scientific lit-erature and the patient's situation). If, for instance, a neurologist for a patient with paralysis prescribes a fancy wheelchair, a utilization review director will discuss the clinical circumstances with the neurologist and then determine if payment for the wheelchair will be authorized, denied, or reduced to a level compatible with an appropriate alternative. This utilization review can occur either prior to the request for the procedure/device (prospective), during a hospitalization (concurrent), or after the service has been delivered or device has been purchased (retrospective). Interpretation of what constitutes medical necessity by the fund distributors and their physician and nursing staff play a large roll in approval and denial rates.

• **Drug formularies:** approved lists of medications that restrict access to high-cost or duplicative medications unless patients are willing to pay extra. Off-patent (many are generic) and medications with negotiated rebates to fund distributors are encouraged over others.

• **Diagnosis-related groups (DRGs):** a standardized inpatient payment system that uses the cost of the average number of days a patient is hospitalized for a specific condition to apply to all patients admitted with that condition. More than six hundred physical conditions have been assigned maximum allowable hospital days (DRGs). For instance, if the number of days in the hospital for 100 patients admitted with stomach ulcers totals 350, the DRG reimbursement rate for the next year would pay the hospital the average amount for exactly 3.5 days of service for every patient with this condition. Many may be discharged in a day, whereas several may stay longer than a month, such as Mrs. Abraham from Chapter 1. If a patient is discharged earlier than 3.5 days, the hospital profits; if treatment is longer, the hospital loses. This procedure discourages hospitals from keeping patients more days in order to enhance profits. The downside is that it can also lead to premature discharge or refusal to care for complex patients (called cherry-picking) in profit-oriented hospitals. Every year, the number of reimbursement days for individual DRGs to each medical facility is adjusted to reflect the new average number of days for the condition, inflation, and modified DRG designations.

The original purpose of managed care was to cut costs, and to this end it remains devoted. In fact, big players in this management game are paid well to do so (Table 3.1). Further, profits do not even account for exorbitant salaries commanded by health plan chief executives and other executive officers, such as Dr. Bill McGuire of United Health Group with annual earnings in excess of $100 million and retirement stock options of $1.6 billion, which are just a cost of doing business. Like well-trained K9s, fund distributors sniff out high-cost areas and attack.

Twenty years of cost-containment strategies focused on access restrictions, benefit limitations, and provider discounts have largely exhausted their cost-saving potential. The momentum to pare costs has now turned to improving patients' responsibility for consumption of health services by shifting decision-making and the initial payment burden to the patient. High-deductible products, such as consumer-driven health savings accounts (HSAs), have far lower monthly premiums than standard policies but require the subscriber to pay a big chunk of health care expenses out of pocket. Relatively new on the market, the verdict on cost-saving effectiveness of these plans is still out.

A recent Harris poll suggested that what looks like gold could very well be pyrite. By putting the initial financial burden directly on the patient, high-deductible policies seem to be doing exactly what they were intended to do. To avoid paying the up-front deductible, many patients will forego seeking medical service and/or filling a prescription (Table 3.2). A lingering question raised

Table 3.1
Health Plan Profits

	2004 3 Q Earnings (in millions of dollars)	2005 3 Q Earnings (in millions of dollars)	Percentage of Revenue Increase
Aetna (2004 includes nonhealth products)	$1,300	$378	14%
Cigna (enrollment down)	$308	$259	(11%)
Health Net (enrollment down; profits up)	$72	$78	3%
Humana	$89	$50	20%
Pacificare Health Systems	$88	$118	23%
United Health Group	$698	$842	14%
WellChoice	$62	$76	13%
WellPoint (largest membership)	$242	$641	138%

Note: As with any business, this summary of Security and Exchange Commission filings for multiple companies confirms that health plans take their share of profits from health service delivery.
Source: Company filings with Security and Exchange Commission, 2005.

Table 3.2
Prescription Adherence by Type of Health Plan Coverage

	Comprehensive	Consumer-driven
Diabetes	85%	76%
Depression	91%	70%
Chronic pain	91%	77%
Arthritis	91%	84%
Heart disease and hypertension	92%	82%
Cholesterol	98%	84%
Asthma	91%	77%
Allergies	93%	77%
Other	83%	75%

Note: New consumer-driven health plans, such as health savings accounts with high deductibles, are having the intended consequence of reducing indiscriminate use of health services, including prescription medications as shown in this 2005 Harris Interactive poll of 1,354 individuals. It remains to be seen whether noncompliance with recommended medications, as is associated with consumer-driven plans, is associated with higher costs and increased illness complications later on.
Source: Adapted from Harris Interactive, Strategic Health Perspectives, 2005.

by the poll is whether the doctor-recommended prescriptions that are not being filled will result in worsened health and even higher patient costs in the future for patients refusing to spend their money for necessary and/or preventive services. For years, we have used noncompliance with medical recommendations as a predictor of poor outcome.

With this repercussion in mind, HSAs could very well create a type of patient similar to the uninsured, the so-called functionally uninsured.[7] Strapped into paying deductibles as high as $2,000 to $7,000 before insurance kicks in will deter many people from seeking early preventive measures. In the long run, preventive care is exactly what has the potential to significantly lower health care costs. Providers are also feeling the pinch because many patients with these plans fail to put money into the HSA and then stiff the doctor for service charges.

Another cost-saving maneuver in the past several years, this one with a brilliant track record, is a shift away from resource-conserving formulas, like utilization management, to health improvement programs, such as disease and case management. These programs have been particularly worthwhile in minimizing expenditures for the small number of high-cost patients with chronic and complex diseases (Figure 3.2).

Disease and case management programs are designed to disseminate health care information to qualifying patients about their diseases and to advise them on how and where to get the most appropriate care in our fragmented health care system.[8] Though the groups that case and disease management vendors target are different, the aim of both is to promote patient self-sufficiency and personal involvement in better treatment of their disease.

Disease management attends to the needs of chronically ill patients by guiding them in locating resource availability for their specific disorder. With early disease

Figure 3.2 Percentage of health care resources used by complex patients.
A small percentage of complex patients, more than half of whom have concurrent physical and mental health/substance-use disorders, utilize the majority of health care services. Claims data in this southwestern health plan demonstrates that 1 percent use a quarter of health resources and 10 percent use two-thirds.

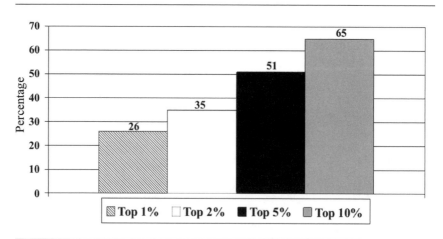

Source: Adapted from R. Kathol and D. Clarke, "Rethinking the Place of the Psyche in Health: Toward the Integration of Health Care Systems," *Australian and New Zealand Journal of Psychiatry* 39 (2005): 816–825.

management intervention, patients suffering from back pain, urinary incontinence, diabetes, hypertension, depression, and other persistent illnesses associated with high costs are more apt to effectively advocate for themselves and follow through on treatment recommendations, thereby whittling total cost while enhancing care. Alvin, the waste management employee from Chapter 1 with asthma/anxiety, would be a perfect candidate for disease management. If Alvin understood the overlap of his illnesses and knew how to navigate the medical system, his plentiful ambulance rides to the emergency room would be substantially curbed.

In addition to disease management, most health plans include more costly but highly valuable case management. This offers assistance to patients with multi-faceted and/or high-cost illnesses that are spinning out of control. Case management usually necessitates active involvement by a medically trained case manager in the intervention process, at least during the period of initial crisis. Depending on the severity of the illness, case managers help primary and specialty caregivers coordinate their efforts with the numerous other participants that influence the patient's progress, such as family members, community services, rehabilitation, ancillary therapies, and so forth.

Repeated hospitalizations for diabetic complications in a patient on dialysis, numerous ER visits, and high levels of health service claims are typical triggers that would invoke case management involvement. Some health plan members receiving disease management, which typically focuses on chronic low-grade illness, are also candidates for case management. If and when an illness takes a turn for the worse, either through nonadherence to good treatment or as a part of the natural course of the illness, the patient would be considered for this service.

Numerous studies document the merits of these assistance programs. As much as $1 to $3 are saved for every dollar spent when patients with common chronic illnesses, such as diabetes, congestive heart failure, end-stage renal disease, or asthma, are enrolled in disease management. Higher returns on health dollars invested in severely ill patients with out-of-control-illnesses are realized when case management teams become involved. Not only do disease and case management services help trim costs, they promote improved health. A novel thought, saving money by improving care! Currently, both purchasers and fund distributors are strong proponents of these services because they consistently promote better clinical outcomes, thus lowering the total cost of health care utilization. Providers and patients, on the other hand, remain skeptical because they have been burned so many times in the past with health plan–generated cost-saving initiatives.

No matter the perpetual endeavor of fund distributors to shore up a crumbling health care system whether by way of the latest HSAs that shift more of the cost burden to the patient or by the introduction of promising assistance programs, mental health and substance-use disorder care remains outside the purview of such innovative enterprises. Early in the transition from fee-for-service to managed care, behavioral health care has been the proverbial elephant in the room.

Almost as soon as managed care was introduced in the early 1980s, special arrangements for the management of behavioral health disorders by fund distributors began. The business stimulus for this was twofold. Psychiatric inpatient stays varied from days to years for patients with the same diagnoses, such as depression. Because of the complex and diverse nature of mental health conditions and, perhaps more importantly, their treatment, assigning average lengths of stay to determine psychiatric DRGs was nearly impossible.

Though long-term insight-oriented psychotherapy in the outpatient setting was on the wane, at least by psychiatrists, it still constituted a major mental health cost with questionable benefit. Those who provided it were, and are, vocal and powerful. As a result, psychiatric care migrated from the managed medical care organizations (MCOs) to discrete managed behavioral health organizations (MBHOs, also commonly referred to as *carve-outs*) in an attempt to allow mental health and substance-use disorder specialists to independently control their own costs.

The best way to understand why MBHOs were considered necessary is to jog back to Eva from Chapter 1, the IT specialist who toppled into a debilitating depression that complicated her diabetes. In the early 1970s, before indemnity insurance gradually gave way to managed care, Eva could have entered two radically different diagnostic and therapeutic approaches for depression: the biological or the insight-oriented psychotherapeutic and all shades in between. Let us look at the extremes.

At that time, insurance guidelines did not require that a mental disturbance had to be "dangerous to protect the patient or society" for a patient to be hospitalized. In fact, treatment in the inpatient setting was less expensive in terms of out-of-pocket costs to the patient than outpatient care because indemnity insurance picked up most inpatient costs. Given these circumstances, it is safe to assume Eva would have been treated for depression in the hospital, at least initially.

Under the biological paradigm, a diagnostic assessment would have first confirmed the presence of a serious major depression disorder. During an average 5- to 14-day admission, Eva would have been treated aggressively with medication in a hospital milieu specifically designed to improve socialization and coping skills and to help her address distressing life issues. Little attention would have been given to her diabetes other than to monitor and prevent medically dangerous blood sugars. In the event of a dip or spike in her glucose levels, a physical health physician would be called.

Upon discharge, Eva would be connected with an outpatient psychiatrist and, perhaps, a psychotherapist if specific life stresses were thought to complicate her clinical picture. By three months, remission and possibly resolution of symptoms would be expected. Eva should be back to her normal self. After hospitalization, clinic visit intervals gradually would decrease from weekly to every other week, then to monthly or bimonthly during the first six months, and occur less frequently thereafter. Her diabetes would remain outside the bounds of her psychiatric treatment.

The experience would have been quite different if Eva were treated using the insight-oriented psychotherapeutic paradigm. Because Eva had good insurance, was intelligent, and possessed good communication skills, she was an ideal candidate for an inpatient admission to a stand-alone psychiatric facility where she would receive individual therapy at least twice a week, if not more. The sessions would focus on traumatic experiences, including sexual abuse, to help Eva gain insight into the underlying early-life events, which led to her breakdown. She would be vaguely diagnosed and a yearlong hospitalization to consolidate the initiation of therapy would be anticipated.

Eva would fill her hospital time with quiet, but helpful, interaction with staff and other patients in an inpatient milieu similar to that of the biological approach; however, the pace of group sessions would be much more relaxed and far from mandatory. Medications would be used sparingly, if at all. Throughout her extended hospital stay, an internist would follow and treat Eva's blood sugar level, if needed, but there would be little interaction with mental health staff.

After discharge, Eva would be scheduled for outpatient therapy sessions twice weekly or more. These might well stretch into years, depending on how the therapist and Eva felt about therapeutic progress. Because the goal of therapy was insight about the underlying cause of her breakdown, symptoms of depression could persist or dissipate without affecting the continued need for inpatient, and eventually outpatient, treatment. Unless there was a risk of suicide, depression would be a peripheral concern.

As illustrated by Eva's clinical situation, behavioral health belt-tightening for service usage was legitimate and long overdue. Almost 10 percent of the total health care dollar in some regions at the time managed care was introduced was devoted to behavioral health care, largely for services to clients with mild illness using treatments with questionable effectiveness. This open-ended and ineffective approach to symptom resolution, plus escalating inflation rates for behavioral health far in excess of general medical care, made it a no-brainer for self-respecting general medical managed health plan administrators to handle behavioral health differently. Thus the era of the MBHO dawned.

One of the first and most influential decisions, which shaped many of the barriers that all patients now face in getting coordinated general medical and behavioral health care, was to create a DRG exemption for psychiatric admissions. Initially, the exemption appeared to be a redemption. Psychotherapeutic programs breathed a sigh of relief that mandated short hospital stays would not be rigidly imposed on behavioral health patients. Gradually, however, the exemption reclaimed the redemption and independently chipped away at excessively long psychiatric hospital stays and non-evidence-based long-term therapies.

With MBHOs also came behavioral health provider networks. The keynote of the behavioral health provider networks is that they essentially severed connection with practitioners in physical health networks and established independent guidelines of operation that included:

- Differentials in physical versus mental health and substance-use disorder benefit restrictions, especially in relation to government programs, such as Medicare (Table 3.3).

Table 3.3
Mental Health Benefit Restrictions by Employer Size

	Small	*Large*	*Total*
Annual inpatient days	58%	67%	64%
Outpatient visits	66%	78%	74%
50% versus 20% co-pay and/or coinsurance	17%	24%	22%

Note: The 2002 Kaiser Family Foundation annual survey documented the percentage of large and small employers that provided their employees with insurance, which restricted annual and lifetime inpatient days and outpatient visits and required a 50 percent rather than a 20 percent co-pay at the time of service for mental health care.
Source: Adapted from Kaiser Foundation Survey, 2002.

- Rigorous behavioral health utilization management practices, far more stringent than physical health utilization criteria.
- Mandated payment rules that behavioral health practitioners work in nonmedical units and clinics or reimbursement schedules that make it impossible to do otherwise.
- Restrictive medication management policies adjudicated solely for psychiatrists.
- Relaxed training and supervision requirements for therapists who provide support and crisis intervention with limited access to therapists with skills in outcome-changing therapies.
- Less expensive partial inpatient and intensive outpatient programs.
- Limits in substance-use disorder treatment to an outpatient setting with rare exceptions.
- Maintenance of an autonomous financial bottom line; that is, physical health and psychiatric services reimbursed from separate buckets of health care dollars.

Reporting on the impact that managed care business practices had on physical and behavioral health care in 1999, the Hay Group documented that the physical health care dollar bought 12 percent less value between 1988 to1998. The behavioral health dollar, however, bought 55 percent less value—a four-and-a-half-fold difference in devaluation.[9]

Close scrutiny of excessive and/or ineffective practices in behavioral health was clearly justified. But, unfortunately, funds that were recaptured over these 10 years of management procedures were not redirected to cover the costs of behavioral health to the 70 percent of patients with psychiatric illness who were receiving no treatment, especially those in the medical sector. Nor was it reallocated to pay for physical health services. So where did it go?

The proceeds from the estimated 7 percent drop in the total health care dollars spent for behavioral health largely went to investor profit at the expense of society at large. Failure to redirect funds for improved mental health and substance-use disorder care, coupled with fragmentation in physical and behavioral health care that MBHOs heralded for patients with psychiatric illness, created a critical and escalating, if not tragic, trajectory in our health care system. At the extreme, today's overcrowded jails with mentally ill patients and a growing population of homeless are stark reminders of how segregating behavioral health has reintroduced the Bedlam-like notion of mental illness as criminal and has reinforced stigmatization for patients in need of mental health treatment.

Since the launch of managed care, fund distributors have tried many things to address excessive health care spending, but, in review, have they really made progress? Administrative costs remain substantial and divert resources from patient care. Despite their efforts, health care costs continue to rise, on average 2.5 percent higher than the annual consumer price index. Although there was a dip in the annual percentage increase in insurance premiums in the mid-1990s (Figure 3.3),[10] this has now reversed. The U.S. population continues to pay considerably more than any other industrialized country.

Providers (Clinicians, Clinics, and Hospitals)

In an ideal world, clinicians would be ethically above reproach, providing excellent care to all patients in exchange for a fair wage. Without prejudice, delivery systems, whether a hospital, rehabilitation center, clinic, or nursing home, would give strong support to clinicians and patients and be justly compensated. Like a well-tuned orchestra, the provider coalition—professionals and facilities—would facilitate diagnosis and treatment, speed responsiveness in crisis, ameliorate suffering, reduce impairment, and go home at night feeling a job well done. This is not an ideal world.

Figure 3.3 Increases in health insurance premiums.
The inflation of health care premiums far outstrips overall inflation in the United States despite monumental attempts to reign in health care costs. Worker salaries parallel general inflation. Health care is on the brink of being unaffordable for all, not just a few.

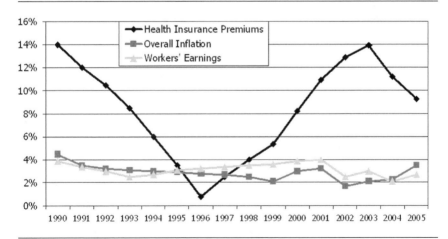

Source: Adapted from Kaiser Family Foundation, "Employer Health Benefits," *Kaiser Family Foundation and Health Research and Educational Trust*, 2005, http://www.kff.org/insurance.

Since the introduction of managed care in the 1980s, providers have been in a pitched battle with health plans to maintain income while attempting to retain quality. Clinicians have largely accomplished income maintenance by seeing more patients during shorter visits and ensuring quality by concentrating on medically acceptable (necessary/evidence-based) assessments and interventions with the greatest financial return. They have been assisted by their hospital and clinic administrators, who outline in black and white the number of patients who need to be seen per hour and the programs that need to be offered to turn a profit while still providing evidence-based quality care. During this process, slowly but exorably, medicine has moved from a helping profession to a business.

The majority of health care clinicians put in long hours and are masters in their selected area of medicine. Most deserve your trust when you bet your life on the care they give. They are also pragmatists and, in general, very bright people. In response to managed care's challenge to lower costs, concessions clearly have been made. Hospital stays have shortened, lower-cost personnel are increasingly used for low-risk or minimally invasive examinations or procedures, and time with patients has become circumscribed. All this has been done with an eye to retaining quality. In fact, many important cost-saving and care-enhancing health processes have been introduced as a result of managed care.

The rub really occurs with the way that the industry has defined cost savings and care quality. Cost savings is invariably expressed in terms of quarterly or annual expense reduction because these are the time lines purchasers use to review expenses as they plan for annual health care contract renewal. Further, budgets are segregated.

There may be great ostensible cost savings in discouraging indiscriminant health care service use by fostering consumer (patient) involvement in decision-making with high deductible insurance products (HSAs) yet an unmeasured loss in terms of worse clinical outcomes, a greater number of emergency room visits, and higher admission rates to hospitals when patients avoid the cost of mammograms, colonoscopies, and/or early clinical evaluations to save money. This does not even take into account the financial impact of days missed from work, poor job performance, and short-term disability payments.

Because it is difficult to measure medical outcomes, especially at the practitioner level, care quality in the managed care environment is typically described in terms of adherence by practitioners in clinical settings to evidence-based medical practices (called *process measures*) rather than to the clinical improvement of their patients. Using this metric, practitioners in a clinic may have an excellent record of blood pressure measurement and antihypertensive medication prescribing, yet fewer then 50 percent of their patients have effectively controlled hypertension (a number commonly found in research studies).

Enhanced health care outcomes require more than just making sure that the patient is on the right medication for an accurately made diagnosis. Many other factors are involved in whether patients get better. Patients also need to understand: (1) the illness and its complications, (2) the importance of adhering to treatment, (3) how to determine if they are responding to treatment, (4) the value of follow-up (especially if the condition is chronic), (5) the desired endpoint, and (6) how to maintain gains. Perhaps more importantly, they must have the resources to pay for evaluations and treatment (medications, etc.) and sufficient intelligence to adhere to treatment recommendations. Because of the inherent physical and/or mental disruption of an illness, many also need transportation to get to clinic and test appointments, a support system that encourages and assists with recovery, adequate time to recuperate, and the motivation to work toward a successful health solution.

Attention to these factors is not built into the current fund distributor-based reimbursement system. Practitioners clearly could choose to regulate clinic visit times to adjust to patient needs and/or set up educational and follow-up programs for complex patients. That choice, however, involves undesirable consequences in terms of fewer reimbursable hours, condescension by fellow practitioners with better patient throughput, deletion from network provider lists, and clinical program dissolution due to insolvency. As a result, side conversations with patients about family, job, and hobbies are limited. There is no time to explain how important adherence is to treatment or what to expect in terms of disease resolution. Most patients have come to expect long waits in doctors' offices, followed by zip-zip and you-are-out evaluations. Doctors, for their part, are spending much more time completing paperwork relative to delivering patient care.

Although clinicians are clearly swayed by the way purchasers and fund distributors define cost savings and care quality, provider facilities are influenced by different challenges. Hospitals and clinics have to make money to survive. To do so, facility administrators direct business development and practices toward medical services that have the most likelihood of financial success. By way of fund distributor reimbursement equations, procedure-oriented programs reap the largest dividends for both professionals and facilities. Cardiology, general and orthopedic surgery, and transplantation are recognized blue-chips in facility portfolios. Less desirable services for facilities to attract and nurture are those with high volume but low-income production, such as family practice, pediatrics, psychiatry, and general internal medicine clinics.

In cases where a health care market has a low percentage of uninsured or underinsured patients, hospitals and clinics and the relatively low-income-generating professionals that treat patients in them still can make a profit. The resources and effort required in locations that serve increasing percentages of poorly insured patients, however, make it much more difficult to do so. Unless subsidized by blue-chip programs or disproportionate share funds, services, such as behavioral health, office-based care management, geriatrics, and even family practice, take on a low priority in decisions about which services to support. To the extent that low-income services can be identified as loss leaders (i.e., they indirectly bring in high-profit patients through a fixed referral network), they rise on the preference list of low-income services to support.

The independent management of behavioral health providers has had intended and unintended consequences. Because it grew out of the need to control inappropriate use of health resources in the specialized behavioral health environment, intended consequences included the isolation and control of mental health and substance-use disorder providers from their physical health colleagues. Only through this mechanism was it considered possible to impact the separately managed and measured behavioral health budget. For practitioners this meant: (1) practicing in geographically and financially segregated provider networks, (2) separate oversight processes and personnel for review of service utilization practices, and (3) success measured in terms of an isolated behavioral health budget reduction. This was done while trying to retain support for evidence-based service, especially to those with severe and persistent mental and substance-use disorders willing to be seen in the circumscribed behavioral health sector.

Behavioral health practitioners were discouraged from practice in the physical health setting, a location in which there would be less control of psychiatric assessment and intervention practices. To accomplish this, management rules required that services be provided in behavioral health inpatient and outpatient locations. When this was considered impossible, rigid prior authorization practices were engaged. In the event authorization was given, low reimbursement for services rendered by credentialed mental health and substance-use disorder clinicians in the physical health setting guaranteed that the number of patients seen in the non-behavioral health sector with behavioral health problems would be limited.

To facilities, independent management of behavioral health translated into isolation of inpatient and/or outpatient mental health and substance-use disorder treatment settings from physical health services, including psychiatric inpatient units, whether in general hospitals or stand-alone structures. It also meant segregated partial hospitalization programs; regular, intensive, and residential outpatient programs; and substance-use disorder programs. Each of these had clearly delineated characteristics, including therapeutic processes and staffing levels that formed the parameters for credentialing and thus reimbursement.

Unintended consequences occurred immediately and then advanced as independently managed behavioral health business practices matured. Perhaps the first and most devastating effect of independent management was practitioner-based abandonment of responsibility and accountability for cross-disciplinary outcomes in the patients they saw. Primary care physicians no longer addressed nor cared about the identification and treatment of depression or anxiety in their patients because it now was supposed to be under the financial and clinical supervision of practitioners in the behavioral health sector.

Psychologists and psychiatrists, likewise, did not see concurrent abdominal bloating, headaches, and dizzy spells in their domain because general medical doctors treated physical symptoms. In fact, as time progressed, practitioners and administrators in both the general medical and behavioral health disciplines became so disconnected with each other that they abandoned any attempts to coordinate services in patients with concurrent illness. It was just too complicated.

Later unintended consequences were more insidious. High-end (and high-cost) behavioral health professionals (i.e., psychiatrists) were forced to "push pills" because this was the one thing that they could do that other mental health and substance-use disorder practitioners could not. Eventually, as budgets were ratcheted down, it was no longer possible for psychiatrists to maintain relationships with the patients they saw during the 15-minute visits mandated by the clinics in which they worked. Even doctoral- and master's-level therapists qualified in evidence-based here-and-now therapies could not make a living due to low levels of reimbursement. Many, in fact, have been replaced by counselors capable only of providing support and crisis intervention—features necessary, but not sufficient, to predictably improve outcomes in patients with psychiatric illness, such as depression and anxiety.

The latest unintended consequence is currently under way. A large number of psychiatrists and psychologists no longer belong to managed behavioral health, Medicare, or Medicaid provider panels. They have had it with the managed care hassles. Rather, they run cash-only practices in which they, not the system, control visit length and intervention capabilities. As a result, the most critically ill and costly patients, most of whose care is managed through a health plan or government agency, can not get access to the very clinicians most able to return them to health. The dwindling few remaining in the mental health and substance-use disorder setting to fulfill the legal-access needs required by the fund distributors are either extremely dedicated and selfless or marginally qualified behavioral health personnel. The latter are incapable of administering treatment that would be essential to resolve psychiatric illness and thus bring little value to their patients or the system.

Patients

Patients are active players in the health care drama, and how successfully they play their part is critical to their own health and the health care system as a whole. After years of practice, it has become apparent that patients fall into four dynamic service-use categories:

- Those who use no services (the abstainers—about 15 percent, including children).
- Those who use occasional services (the hale and hearty—about 75 percent).
- Those without serious illness who frequently use services (the illness worriers).
- Those with serious illness who frequently use services (the ill).

The last two categories and a small component of the hale and hearty who suffer catastrophic events make up only 10 percent of the population, but they use a startling 65 percent of health resources (Figure 3.2)! Although patients will fall into and out of these categories based on changing clinical situations, the percentages hold remarkably stable.

The abstainers are usually inheritors of a strong gene pool and are more likely to be seen at a yoga retreat or a walkathon than in a pharmacy. They get periodic checkups and preventive screening tests, maintain a healthy weight, and exercise regularly. Very few of them are addicted to tobacco or doughnuts.

The hale and hearty, averaging one to four outpatient visits per year with no more than one short hospital admission every five to eight years, constitute the majority of individuals in our health care system. They use the system for preventive or corrective measures but do not warrant significant monitoring. Sixty percent to 80 percent in this category will be seen from time to time by their general practitioners for unexplained physical complaints, such as weakness, insomnia, shoulder pain, dizziness, and so forth. More often than not, minor assessment and reassurance resolves their health concerns. Included in this group are also those with stress, personal or family crises, life-phase issues, and so forth. Although needing attention, symptoms are transient. Patients get over them and go about their business.

Frequent users tap the bulk of health care resources and demand closer attention for both clinical and economic reasons. Included in this category are patients with catastrophic illness (the ill) who may be in need of an organ transplant or care for extensive accident-related injuries. It is usually a one-time hit, but an extended and very expensive hit. Also falling into this category is the group of patients who suffer with chronic general medical illnesses, such as diabetes, end-stage kidney disease, multiple sclerosis, asthma, emphysema, cystic fibrosis, heart failure, and so forth, and chronic and/or recurrent psychiatric illnesses such as schizophrenia, autism, bipolar affective disorder, or anorexia.

These chronic general medical and psychiatric conditions are pretty straightforward. The patients require good evidence-based care and benefit from case and disease management services. If well educated about the nature of their illness and motivated by their care providers, they can be influenced to take the initiative to adhere to treatment recommendations and seek help before expensive crises erupt. With guidance from case or disease managers (almost exclusively restricted to patients with general medical illness in today's system), they also are better equipped to navigate the health care system and more wisely use their health care dollars.

The illness worriers, of which a significant portion are patients with untreated or ineffectively treated psychiatric illness, are possibly the most challenging segment counted in the population of frequent users. This group has habitual and recurrent symptoms without identifiable physical causes. Characteristically, they have a high sensitivity to suggestion. Josef Babinski, a neurologist at the turn of the century, called the condition *pithiatism*,[11] explaining that symptoms can be "caused by suggestion and cured by persuasion." Normal, yet variable, mental processes magnify minor complaints to the extent that the person experiencing the symptoms is convinced a serious illness is afoot and goes straight to a doctor for evaluation.

Instead of offering simple reassurance that all is well, doctors are compelled to test, medicate, and refer, which can, and often does, put the patient at risk.[12] Adverse events and complications do occur from excessive testing and treatment, such as allergic reactions and medication side effects. In this sense, illness worriers and their doctors end up being the greatest health threat. With concern over medical lawsuits, however, doctors have had to become overly cautious. Rather than trust their gut instincts, they often opt to cover their posteriors with reams of test results.

In the movie *Field of Dreams,* Ray Kinsella heard a voice, "If you build it, he will come." My experience with the relatively small percentage that are illness worriers is that "If these patients hurt, they will come." They will come often and to many clinicians searching for the magic that will douse their health concern, much as we saw with Margie in Chapter 1. They will be given one test after another, and more than one too many pill bottles will line their medicine cabinets. Interestingly, in patients with an underlying psychiatric condition, such as anxiety or depression, failure to recognize and treat it to remission perpetuates the cycle of test-refer-treat for unexplained physical complaints and leads to the well-documented high total cost of care.

This group particularly highlights the insanity of the behavioral health carve-out in which perception of bodily processes, not physical illness, leads to high service utilization and explosive costs if not appropriately addressed and treated. Furthermore, if more than two-thirds of health care costs are generated by fewer than 10 percent of patients, as the numbers indicate, then those who use the majority of services will quickly surpass even a high deductible. The incentive they may have had to conserve resources prior to meeting health savings account deductible limits will then disappear, and the bank's safe opens.

OVERLAP OF GENERAL MEDICAL AND BEHAVIORAL DISORDERS

In Chapter 2 we discussed the medical and psychiatric illness interaction, but most do not realize the frequency with which this occurs. Concurrent and clinically significant psychiatric symptoms coexist in more than a fourth of patients with general medical conditions (Table 3.4). Many studies of depression in the medical setting underscore this relationship. For instance, diabetes, asthma,

Table 3.4
Prevalence of Mental Disorders in Nonpsychiatric Settings

	Community Setting	Primary Care Setting	General Hospital Admission
Major depression	5.1%	5%–14%	>15%
Somatization	0.2%	2.8%–5%	2%–9%
Substance abuse	6.0%	10%–30%	20%–50%
Any disorder	18.5%	21%–26%	30%–60%

Note: This summary of clinical studies demonstrates that mental health and substance-use disorders are seen with increasing prevalence as one moves from community samples to outpatient general medical clinics to general medical inpatient units.
Source: Adapted from Cole et al., Task Force on Health Care Value Enhancement, 1997.

heart disease, stroke, cancer, to name a few, are all associated with a 20 percent to 40 percent prevalence of depression.

Although the most common mental health problem seen in a nonpsychiatric setting today is depression, other emotional, cognitive, and behavioral presentations also occur with greater frequency in the physical health setting, such as anxiety, eating disorders, substance-use disorders, somatic complaints, dementia, delirium, and even psychoses. Most of these patients are exclusively under the care of nonpsychiatrist physicians, many of whom lack the training to evaluate and treat psychiatric disorders. When poor training is coupled with administrative and payment mandates absolving them of the responsibility to effectively treat mental health and substance-use disorders, it is no surprise that general medical patients with comorbid psychiatric illness have much worse clinical and economic outcomes (Table 3.5).[13]

For many patients treated in the medical setting, little attention is given to hidden or even manifest psychiatric symptoms. The reverse is equally true for a large percentage of physically ill patients seen in the psychiatric setting. Several studies now show that many common physical conditions are frequent in patients with mental health and substance-use disorders. Patients with anxiety and/or depression are nearly twice as likely to have asthma than patients who do not. In fact, patients with severe and persistent mental illness, such as schizophrenia or bipolar illness, have exceptionally high levels of medical illness (Table 3.6).[14]

Characteristically, psychiatric patients do not advocate well for themselves. Fewer than half have a primary care physician, and those who do find it difficult or uncomfortable to access physical health services. Unable to qualify and/or pay for private insurance, they are usually enrollees in low-reimbursement public programs like Medicaid and have financial worries that contribute to their reluctance to seek help.

The vestiges of stigma attached to mental health and substance-use disorders also are pronounced roadblocks, not only among the patients suffering with mental illness but also within the circle of those trying to manage their care. By assigning a completely separate system to handle mental illness, the stigma is perpetuated. It is

Table 3.5
Health Care Utilization by General Medical Patients

	DM, CV, HT, and BP	Depressed Only	Depressed and Ill
	(N = 1,956)	(N = 312)	(N = 100)
Health care cost	$3,853	$3,417	$7,407
Sick days	6.64	8.79	13.48
Per capita health and disability costs	$4,646	$4,675	$7,906

Note: The research findings reported by Druss et al. show that depression itself is as incapacitating and costly as diabetes mellitus (DM), cardiovascular illness (CV), hypertension (HT), and back pain (BP), but when co-occurring with these physical illnesses it more than doubles human suffering and the financial toll.
Source: Adapted from B. G. Druss, R. A. Rosenheck, and W. H. Sledge, "Health and Disability Costs of Depressive Illness in a Major U.S. Corporation," *American Journal of Psychiatry* 157, no. 8 (August 2000): 1274–78.

assumed that having mental illness is so special that it cannot be treated with the rest of medical conditions. Though a wide variety of health professionals in the non-psychiatric setting regularly and openly address sensitive and private conditions like erectile dysfunction and unwanted pregnancies, bipolar illness or drug addiction remain untouchables.

The documented high frequency with which general medical illness interacts with psychiatric illness poses a couple of critical questions. To what advantage do we separate general medical and psychiatric care at a time when the demand for mental health care is at an all-time high? And are behavioral health specialists and general medical specialists willing to work together to improve care for comorbid patients to eliminate the disadvantages of not doing so?

We will see how independently managed behavioral health care plays out in the next chapter and how fragmentation of the health care infrastructure is the problem, not the solution. Autonomous physical health and behavioral health business and clinical practices prevent smooth, effective, and financially sound coordination of health care. As long as this type of health care system persists, patients like Eva, Mohammed, and Harry will continue to jump through hoops trying to get integrated care or die prematurely and unnecessarily from either complications of an ineffectively treated medical condition or suicide related to poorly treated psychiatric illness.

The body *and* mind function as a unit. To approach treatment of either in isolation is a disservice to those suffering with comorbid conditions and a financial catastrophe to those who have to pay for it. Personal interaction historically has been invaluable in healing both body and mind, but in our current system the personal element

Table 3.6
Prevalence of Medical Disorders in Patients with Severe and Persistent Mental Illness

	Prevalence
Pulmonary	31%
Heart	22%
Gastrointestinal	25%
Skin and connective tissue	19%
Metabolic	15%
Diabetes	12%
Any medical illness	75%
Two or more medical illnesses	50%

Note: Severely and persistently mentally ill patients have very high rates of medical illness. Despite the fact that 75 percent have at least one medical illness and a half have more than one, these patients find it difficult to access medical services.
Source: Adapted from D. R. Jones, C. Macias, P. J. Barreira, W. H. Fisher, W. A. Hargreaves, and C. M. Harding, "Prevalence, Severity, and Co-occurrence of Chronic Physical Health Problems of Persons with Serious Mental Illness," *Psychiatric Services* 55, no. 11 (2004): 1250–57.

has vanished. Transferring policy decisions to health plan administrators, with profit motives no less robust than the providers they control, has mutated the practice of medicine into a processing plant.

Looking back, it probably would have been better for all involved just to give lower, yet fixed, wages to doctors, hospitals, and clinics and to allow them to provide services in the way they considered most appropriate and effective. As it is, the clinical component of the medical system of today resembles that of our failing education system in which administration, with an inflexible set of rules, unsuccessfully tries to run the classroom.

Chapter 4

MANGLED MEDICINE

As to diseases make a habit of two things—to help, or at least, to do no harm.[1]

—Hippocrates

A HEALTH SYSTEM IN DISARRAY

No fictitious scare tactic about it. There is a bogeyman under the bed, and it is the U.S. health care system. In 2005, health insurance premiums increased more than 9 percent—nearly three times the rate of inflation (Figure 3.3).[2] Forty-six million Americans are uninsured.[3] Out-of-pocket health care spending rose $13.7 billion to an astounding $230 billion in 2003.[4] Although the overall inflation rate has held steady at 2 percent to 4 percent between 1990 and 2005, health care inflation has yo-yoed between 0.8 percent and 18 percent. Family annual health premiums have risen from $4,024 to $10,881, with no projected stabilization in sight.

Despite rigorous, if not draconian, cost-saving efforts by health plans, the cost of care continues to rise at unacceptable rates. Whether privately insured or in publicly financed programs, like Medicare and Medicaid, most people are intimately familiar with some of the more common management cost-controlling practices. To name a few: different rates for tiered providers, long waits on the telephone to obtain prior approval for tests or referrals, and restrictions on medications through health plan formularies.

At 15 percent of the gross domestic product (GDP), the United States spends more on health care than do other industrialized nations, including countries that provide health insurance to all their citizens. Health costs in the United States are nearly a third more than in Switzerland, the next highest priced national health system at 11.5 percent of the GDP, and health outcomes are no better. In many instances, they are worse than other developed nations, partly because emphasis on acute care trumps preventive care in a system driven by misplaced competition.

Michael Porter and Elizabeth Teisberg, in the June 2004 issue of *Harvard Business Review,* cogently argue that one of the major reasons that the health system in the United States has performed so poorly is that health plan–based management creates zero-sum competition.[5] Using the zero-sum approach, the health care industry competes with a focus on reducing costs rather than driving up value, as would be found with positive-sum competition. This happens in several ways:

- It shifts costs from one player to another, such as payer to patient (health savings accounts), health plan to hospital (utilization review), uninsured to insured (no universal participation), state budget to federal budget and back (Medicaid), and so forth.

- It attempts to get better contract bargains while giving no better than lip service to quality, efficiency, and outcomes.

- It restricts the choice of doctors, clinics, hospitals, medications, and so on and access to selected treatments and services through benefit descriptions, provider networks, and medication formularies based ostensibly on quality but actually on negotiated reimbursement rates.

- It relies on a capricious court system to arbitrate disputes.

Only loosely interested in long-term health improvement, zero-sum competition emphasizes quarterly or annual savings on budget segments, whereas positive-sum competition stresses competition on quality at the care-delivery and disease-outcome levels. Further, positive-sum competition uses total long-term health care costs as its economic success metric. When focusing competition on the quality of care, providers that bring clinical, functional, and economic value through superior patient outcomes receive the majority of health care business.

The Institute of Medicine's document *Crossing the Quality Chasm: A New Health System for the 21st Century (Chasm Report)* targets quality of care provisions from the patient's perspective as the driving force for change rather than business practices.[6] In contrast, Porter and Teisberg approach the health care crisis from a business perspective. Indeed, it is important that the health system aim to make health care safe, effective, patient-centered, timely, efficient, and equitable as the *Chasm Report* encourages. To ensure viability, vitality, and longevity, however, the financial health care infrastructure must be organized so that the quality measures described in the *Chasm Report* can be realized.

To change the formula from zero-sum to positive-sum competition, the authors contend fundamental changes must occur (Table 4.1).

Positive-sum competition would adopt universal participation in health coverage and emphasize transparency of provider experience, clinical success, and price of care. To maintain a solid community reputation and patient base, providers would need to emulate clinical and organizational practices that lead to healthier patients

Table 4.1
Features of Positive-Sum Competition

No restrictions on competition and choice
For example:
  No network limits
  No preapprovals
  Strict antitrust enforcement
  Meaningful co-pays and/or high deductibles
Accessible information
For example:
  On treatment alternatives
  On provider experience, cost, and success (report cards)
  On benchmarks
Transparent pricing
For example:
  A single price for a given treatment available to patients before the treatment is given
Simplified billing
For example:
  Single hospital and episode-of-illness billing with quick reimbursement to providers
Nondiscriminatory insurance
For example:
  Required universal participation with a national risk pool for all accepted services and
  procedures
Treatment coverage
For example:
  Required basic with buy-up capabilities for additional coverage
Fewer lawsuits
For example:
  Better informed consent
  Expert review of cases for evidence of negligence prior to suit
  Built-in monitoring for unsafe providers

Note: Porter and Teisberg describe suggested changes needed to drive the health system from zero-sum competition, which focuses on cost, to positive-sum competition, which focuses on value. Misplaced competition perpetuates high cost and poor outcomes.
Source: Adapted from Michael Porter and Elizabeth Teisberg, "Redefining Competition in Health Care," *Harvard Business Review* 82, no. 6 (June 2004): 65–76.

in an atmosphere of ready access to the cost of services. Transparency would give patients the ability to make decisions about the use of more expensive providers where they likely would get treatment resulting in better prevention and/or control of illness and ultimately lower overall and long-term cost. Patients, in the positive-sum scenario, given the opportunity to shop around for the best value, also would invigorate healthy competition and inspire excellence.

Sorely missing in our health care system today is a transparent, comprehensive price list. In any other consumer-driven area, whether it is shopping for clothes or a bottle of wine, consumers can relate quality to cost. Depending on the motivation of the purchaser, one may choose to buy hiking boots at REI and rubber flip-flops at Wal-Mart. If Safeway is selling salmon for $4.99 per pound, and the corner market has it at $7.99 per pound, motivated by price or convenience, the consumer makes the choice where to buy the salmon. Health is a high priority for most people, and yet the quality-price ratio is shrouded in mystery when it comes to clinics, hospitals, clinician services, medications, labs, X-rays, and medical supplies.

In Minnesota, a 2004 law requires that clinics provide good-faith estimates of what a patient will pay for services. The patient, however, has to work hard for these estimates. After months on the telephone with hospital and clinic system business offices as well as with my reluctant health plan, a comparison of five major provider groups revealed that clinic charges for a physical health screening evaluation (examination, EKG, chest X-ray, mammogram) with basic labs (blood count, occult blood, prostate antigen, lipids, metabolic screen) and one follow-up visit ranged from $645 to $1,040. For insured persons, the comparative costs ranged from $427 to $959 after health plan discounts.

If screening colonoscopy is needed, differences in costs are even more impressive. Doctor charges ranged from $626 to $1,260 and the procedure room from $809 to $1,761. Health plan–based discounts from the amounts charged by the clinics for professional and facility fees were from 10 percent to 49 percent of charges. Thus professional and facility fees for those with health plan coverage ranged from $536 to $1,134 and $625 to $1,526, respectively. An uninsured patient could spend anywhere from $1,487 to $2,955 and, if insured, from $1,196 to $2,660 for the same preventive evaluation with colonoscopy—a $1,468 to $1,464 difference in price, respectively. Quality indicators were nowhere to be found, and it took three months on the phone with long waits to complete the comparisons.

In most states, price information is proprietary and, therefore, not available. Even in Minnesota, where by law it is required to provide the information, it was necessary to seek the assistance of the attorney general's office to get some of the clinic groups to share their charges and the discounted (allowed) amounts that the health plan paid to them. Without this information, patients have no way of knowing what potential savings are available, let alone whether those that charge more provide extra clinical value. Further, hiding such information takes away any incentive for providers to curb their own charges. Lack of transparency completely defeats the purpose of a consumer-driven health plan (CDHP, also known as a health savings account, or HSA).

Porter and Teisberg's positive-sum competition strategy is one of many financial blueprints being floated to correct the ills of a broken system, but the question of when purchasers of health insurance might expect to see relief from rapidly rising health care costs and insurance premiums remains a perennial one.[7] Paul Ginsburg, president of the Center for Studying Health System Change, wrote in an article for *Health Affairs* that "If health care spending continues to grow at a significantly faster rate than workers' incomes—and there's every sign that it will—health insurance will become unaffordable to more and more people."[8] The fewer people paying into the system, the less funding there is to run the system, and the decline of quality health care will accelerate.

Without a major overhaul, this dismal situation can only get worse. Beginning in 2006, an estimated 78 million boomers celebrated 60th birthdays at a rate of 7,900 every single day, and they are expected to live longer than any other previous U.S. generation![9] As these rock and rollers "rage, rage against the dying of the light,"[10] our current health care system will topple under the load. Profound steps must be taken, which include, but are not limited to:

- Citizens (patients) must accept that universal health coverage for basic health care benefits is required for quality to improve and for cost controls to work. This is not synonymous with a single-payer paradigm that strikes loathing in many American hearts that cannot imagine big government playing God. Many countries with uniform universal national coverage do not operate in a single-payer format. Many have numerous social insurance companies that foster healthy competition and meet specific areas of need. In France, three separate companies administer so-called sickness funds, 300 operate in Germany, and more than 5,000 are up and running in Japan. All operate at substantially less cost per citizen than do those in the United States. Individuals, who need or want coverage for services in excess of basic national benefits can purchase supplements depending on their personal situations. They have surpassed the United States in both cost stability and citizen accessibility. Many, in fact, also have healthier populations, suggesting better care.

- Legislators must be willing to regulate selected components of the health care industry, such as pharmaceutical, medical device, and procedure delivery companies offering high-cost components. Among the regulated are designer drugs, gene sequences, antibiotic-impregnated catheters, Cadillac wheelchairs, magnetic resonance imaging (MRI), and positron-emission tomography (PET) scans in order to limit monopoly-like profits that divert resources away from basic care to a larger percentage of the population. For instance, in Japan the average cost of a computerized tomography (CT) scan of the head is $125 compared to $900 to $1,500 in the United States, a 7- to 12-fold difference. Differences in price for MRIs are even more impressive, $160 in Japan and $1,725 to $2,500 in the United States, an 11- to 16-fold difference. An average 90-day supply of 40 milligrams of Lipitor (atorvastatin calcium, an anticholesterol agent) costs $180 in Canada and $310 in the United States.

- Coverage must be consolidated so that all Americans are insured at reasonable premium rates for a defined benefit set. Health care is something far different from electronics. If a person does not have the money to buy an iPod, he or she will think twice before buying it. Not so with health care. Individuals without health insurance, whether they have the money or not, will show up in emergency rooms and on hospital units and they will be treated. It is the law. As mentioned in the previous chapter, in order to keep the practitioners and facilities operating, we will all pay for the care of these individuals in one form or another. If there were but a handful of uninsured individuals, the situation would be far less critical. But there are many, and, typically, they use the highest-cost services for ailments that could have been treated much less expensively in more appropriate medical settings. As well, if they had carried insurance, they probably would have sought intervention prior to requiring much more expensive crisis care. With everyone insured, as would be the case with universal coverage, better clinical outcomes and lower costs are easily predictable.

- Our legislators also must be willing to offer solutions to the public for adverse events that occur through provider negligence other than litigation. These solutions both should prevent future episodes of negligence by unethical or unskilled health care providers (hospitals, clinics, and their practitioners) and should assure that a high percentage of the money paid in damages goes to patients, not to their lawyers.

- Providers, including clinicians, clinics, hospitals, and residential facilities, must allow documentation and publication of the value they bring to the people they treat as well as the associated costs. Although measuring performance is never easy, system sophistication has advanced sufficiently at least to compare clinics and hospitals on major health parameters, and in some instances, it can compare clinicians offering the service. Health care delivery systems have to be willing to measure and give performance feedback to the physicians and other health professionals who staff their clinical settings, adjusting for the severity of illness of the patients so that meaningful comparisons can be made.

- Health plans must become transparent regarding their cost and reimbursement structures. Coverage must be transportable from one plan to another and from state to state. The purchase of coverage must be simplified and have a uniform basic benefit package. Business and management practices must focus on a balance of short- and long-term clinical and financial goals. The information technology infrastructure must be capable of documenting and reporting clinical and financial outcomes. They must work in concert with other management organizations involved in maximizing health, such as disease management, disability management, health promotion, and employee assistance vendors. In short, health plans must become partners with other management vendors and the providers they support rather than adversaries. They also must be accountable for outcomes of the products that they sell.

- Purchasers can not be expected to be familiar with what constitutes value when they buy health care products for their employees, their constituents, or themselves. On the other hand, they can perform on-site reviews, which confirm that the work processes they bought, such as benchmarked case and disease management, are being delivered. They must demand reports that document value as a part of their health plan contracts. A portion of every health care contract must be devoted to effectiveness assessment occurring at both the macro- and micro-outcome levels.

THE PHYSICAL AND BEHAVIORAL HEALTH ILLNESS DISCONNECT

Up to this point, we have skimmed the problems associated with the general medical side of the health care equation, which could keep us busy for some time. It is, however, the contention of this book that unless issues related to mental health and substance-use disorders are shuffled into health care reform discussions, little progress will ensue. The most complex and costly patients, many of whom are uninsured, will continue to receive inadequate and ineffective general medical and psychiatric services, and the financial engine of the system will carry the burden.

Without relying on percentages, tables, and graphs to detail the inadequacies of our current carved-out system of health care, Kathy will put a face on it. She is 53 years old. Her retirement savings are nearly wiped out. Medical bankruptcy is at the door. She is stuck in Virginia, 1,550 miles away from her family, and unable to get coordinated health care for an unexpected and, in many ways, unnecessary collapse of her health. This was not the harvest Kathy intended for herself.

A divorced mother of two, Kathy supported her family by operating an accounting business out of her home and working part-time as a receptionist for Best Buy Realty. When her children left for college, she returned to the University of North Dakota and earned a master's degree in English, graduating with honors. Itching to spread her wings and no longer bound by the constraints of raising kids, she sold her home in Grand Forks and nested the proceeds in an investment fund that would provide for her old age. Always fascinated with colonial American history, Kathy hoped to write a historical novel about the life of Mary Ball Washington, George Washington's mother. With this dream in mind, she moved to Irvington, Virginia, where she rented a small cabin off one of the rural tidewater roads with a spectacular view of the Rappahannock River. She got a part-time job with the Lancaster County Public School District. The combined resources of her salary and a modest dividend from her investments would cover the essentials. If she lived simply, she could live comfortably on her salary and the dividend. Fiercely independent, Kathy looked forward to the solo adventure. And an adventure it would be.

The health insurance plan Kathy had through Best Buy Realty in North Dakota did not follow her to Virginia, and the Irvington school district did not offer health insurance to part-time employees. Like ordering utilities or finding an honest car mechanic, she knew that arranging for health insurance was going to be a pain. Knowing little more about the matrix of health insurance than what she picked up in conversations with coworkers or watching TV talk shows, Kathy was not a savvy health insurance purchaser. She did know, however, that the cleaner her medical records were, the better her chances were of qualifying for a comprehensive and affordable policy. To this end, she had been militant to the extreme.

To the public eye, Kathy's medical record was unremarkable: two normal pregnancies, no surgeries, a benign breast lump, and an adolescent congenital kidney disease (polycystic kidneys). Also included in her open medical history were several bouts with mild depression for which her general internist had long ago prescribed a maintenance dose of the antidepressant Effexor (venlafaxine).

Kathy also was well versed on the inequities in behavioral and general health coverage. Because the health plan Best Buy Realty had purchased for its employees subcontracted their behavioral health management to a company separate from the one that managed the medical side, Kathy's coverage for depression had been nearly nonexistent. By buying insurance from a major, rather than a regional, health company, she hoped to avoid these incongruities. Bigger company, better coverage, she reasoned.

After tedious attempts at comparison shopping and a couple of application denials, Kathy found herself limited to one of two options. She qualified for a Blues plan that carried a price tag of $730 per month.[11] Inquiring about the reasons behind such a costly premium, she learned that it was not related to the benign breast lump, even though her mother had died of breast cancer. Nor was it related to the congenital kidney disease because it had been, expectedly, written out of the policy as a preexisting condition. Rather, the information she reported regarding mild depression sent the rate into orbit.

Her remaining option was a high-deductible health savings account (HSA) priced at $430 per month, which again excluded the polycystic kidney condition. The same policy, without a history of depression, would have cost her $220 per month, but given the subscriber guidelines of most other insurance companies, Kathy was told she was lucky the Blues considered her insurable at all.

For Kathy, the decision was not difficult. A $730 per month premium was out of reach—a budget buster. She signed up for the HSA.

The policy afforded a couple of advantages but, to her mind, hardly compensation. If she kept the $2,500 annual deductible in a savings account earmarked solely for health expenses, what she did not use in one year would accumulate year to year. Provider discounts, also known as *allowed amount deductions,* contracted by the health plan administrators with physician groups, clinics, and hospitals, also would decrease provider charges somewhat. Although this helped her stay below the deductible limit, Kathy had no way to leverage this because charges and allowed amounts were considered proprietary. The money Kathy put away in the account would be tax-deductible, though that particular advantage did not really apply to her financial situation.

An advocate of preventive care, it was Kathy's custom to schedule a physical exam every year on her birthday. From the list of preferred providers included in her plan, she attempted to do so but could not find one nearby doctor in her network that did not have a two-month waiting list. Finally, she made an appointment with a nurse practitioner in Richmond, who was available to see her within a couple of weeks and at a lower cost.

The nurse practitioner and Kathy hit it off right away. A bookworm herself, Lynn was enchanted with Kathy's writing efforts, and being a native of Irvington she had much to contribute about the history of the Chesapeake Bay area. Kathy felt comfortable in Lynn's care, and Lynn did her job well. She recorded Kathy's temperature and weight normal. There were no unusual swellings in her lymph nodes, breasts, or stomach. Reflexes firing, ears clear. With the exception of a blood pressure of 140/95 and an occasional increase in urination, Kathy appeared to be in good health. Lynn started her on a water pill (thiazide diuretic) to stabilize the elevated blood pressure and wrote an order for a mammogram, along with other tests she considered important for a patient with a familial kidney disease.

Lynn was not aware of Kathy's episodes of depression until the end of the exam when Kathy asked for a refill of her Effexor and lithium. Running behind schedule, Lynn quickly wrote a prescription for a month's supply and had Kathy sign a permission form to obtain her medical records from Grand Forks. She made a mental note to herself to ask Kathy additional questions about her medications at the follow-up appointment.

Lynn's initial evaluation of Kathy's health was considered routine until screening laboratory tests came back a week later with microscopic blood in the urine and a twice-normal white blood count. The test results also indicated a creatinine clearance that put Kathy at stage three out of five for chronic kidney disease (creatinine level of 1.6 mg/dl with a calculated half normal clearance [51.4 ml/min]). According to the general medical records that had arrived from the internist in Grand Forks, Kathy's kidney function had not been tested in the last five years. Lynn's concern spiked.

She noted from the records that Kathy's doctor had suggested counseling because of "numerous somatic concerns" for which workups were negative, and treatment nearly always resolved the symptoms within days only to have other symptoms appear. Refills for Effexor were regularly noted, but nothing about lithium. The records did not mention depression, let alone the type of depressive symptoms Kathy had experienced in the medical notes, nor was a counselor's name included. Because psychiatric records were handled separately from general medicine, Lynn had no way of accessing Kathy's mental health records without first locating a clinician's name.

Because lithium was excreted through the kidneys, Lynn was aware that its use in a patient with kidney disease was a potential disaster. Prior to their scheduled follow-up appointment, Lynn called Kathy to the office to discuss the presence of blood in Kathy's urine. Because Kathy had no history of urinary tract infections or any other suspicious reasons for kidney changes, Lynn wanted an ultrasound done to better ascertain if cysts in her kidneys were contributing to Kathy's loss in function. Also, to allay a needling concern about possible adverse drug reactions, she wanted to learn more about Kathy's depression and subsequent treatment.

Lynn's casual probing uncovered that Kathy had well-kept secrets about her mental health. With a family history of mania and depression (bipolar illness), Kathy had been under the care of a Grand Forks psychiatrist for counseling and medication. Over time, to control hypomanic episodes and to avoid potential hospitalization for mania, given Kathy's well-known family history, her psychiatrist, Dr. Dorothy, had added the inexpensive drug lithium to Kathy's Effexor, and for years the combination had maintained her mental health. To keep her psychiatric history off her health plan medical records, Kathy had always paid Dr. Dorothy in cash.

By the time Kathy concluded her story, Lynn realized the clinical situation was much more complicated than she thought and potentially dangerous. She asked Kathy to sign a standard release to obtain the records from Dr. Dorothy and urged Kathy to have an ultrasound and a lithium level. Responding to red flags outside of her expertise, she advised Kathy to schedule an emergency appointment with the clinic's general internist, Dr. Jerome, as well as with a psychiatrist. Mentally calculating the prohibitive expense, Kathy hesitated.

"This could be serious," Lynn said. "Trust me, something isn't right."

Before Kathy was able to see Dr. Jerome, a neighbor brought her into the emergency room. Trembling and confused, incontinent, weak, uncoordinated, speech slurred (dysarthria), Kathy was unable to communicate her distress to the intake nurse. The neighbor explained that they had spent the day at a crab bake and that Kathy had gradually felt "out of control." Asked about alcohol, the neighbor said Kathy did not like beer and had instead tapped the lemonade keg all day.

Emergency room staff quickly stabilized Kathy, packed her into an ambulance, and sent her to St. Mary's in Richmond, which had a better equipped and staffed emergency facility.

A review of the clinic notes revealed a slightly elevated lithium level (1.5 mEq/l) from a test drawn the morning of Kathy's last visit with Lynn, 10 hours after her last dose of lithium. The emergency room doctor immediately ordered a lithium level, and within an hour the results came back four times the therapeutic maximum. All medications were stopped, and Kathy was admitted to St. Mary's Hospital.

Meeting Kathy for the first time, Dr. Jerome recognized the symptoms of lithium intoxication and was aware from his discussions with Lynn that kidney impairment was likely the culprit. Her kidneys were not filtering the lithium, and quick elimination was crucial to avoid permanent nerve damage. He ordered dialysis to rid her body of the excess lithium. After reviewing the medical records, he deduced that an interaction of the water pill Lynn had given to control high blood pressure and Kathy's gradually failing kidneys due to her inherited polycystic disease produced the toxic lithium level. Dehydration on a hot summer day was enough to precipitate the crisis.

During the initial days of hospitalization, Kathy was sleepy but cooperative. On the sixth day, however, her condition took a nosedive. She became demanding, hypertalkative, and grandiose. Pulling out her intravenous line, she refused her third, and last, dialysis and demanded to leave the hospital.

"I feel fine," she said to the congregation of nurses trying to regain control. "Give me my clothes!" Frantically, she tore off her hospital gown and, failing to find her own clothes, fled the intensive care unit butt-naked.

After a tangle of hysterics, security escorted her back to her bed. A stat psychiatry consultation was called, and she was restrained in her bed "for her own safety" until help arrived. Help, however, did not arrive for more than 24 hours because there was no psychiatrist in Kathy's behavioral health insurance network who had privileges at St. Mary's Hospital. Finally, Dr. Bob, a network psychiatrist for Kathy's carve-out but an out-of-network doctor for St. Mary's, was called and assessed the situation after getting permission to see Kathy as a noncredentialed St. Mary's provider.

Predictably, many bipolar patients will have an acute episode of mania when a mood stabilizer, such as lithium, is suddenly discontinued. Dr. Bob suggested trying Zyprexa (olanzapine), a new antimanic agent that had an intramuscular and sublingual preparation if Kathy refused a pill. He counseled the medical staff that Kathy had a right to refuse treatment unless she either was considered dangerous or was officially committed and required to comply with treatment. In fact, because Kathy was being restrained, he suggested she be committed to the unit immediately.

Dr. Bob already had called the psychiatry unit at St. Mary's. They refused to take responsibility for Kathy on the grounds that the behavioral health carve-out had consistently denied reimbursement for services provided to their so-called covered lives in their nonnetwork psychiatry unit. Nor could she be discharged from St. Mary's and transferred to the psychiatric unit at Methodist Hospital, Dr. Bob's network hospital, because she was considered medically unstable. The psychiatric nursing staff at Methodist felt unqualified treating acute mania in a patient with renal insufficiency. Too many complications were likely to arise that would put her recovery in jeopardy, and their tails in the ringer. Plus, they already had a four-person waiting list for the next bed.

Blanks in Kathy's psychiatric history did not expedite treatment. Her records from the psychiatrist in Grand Forks arrived a month after her admission to St. Mary's. They had been delayed by the requirement of a signed nonstandard behavioral health release form and then by Kathy's abnormal mental state at the time the release form became available for her to sign. Also impeding expediency was the demand for reimbursement by the Grand Forks office before the records would be copied and sent. In part, the delay related to the disconnect between the medical and behavioral system and, in part, to Dr. Dorothy's prior agreement with Kathy to protect her psychiatric history from her insurers.

A review of Dr. Dorothy's records revealed that Kathy had a strong family history of bipolar illness and nearly had been hospitalized on several occasions. The combination of lithium and Effexor, along with half-hour supportive therapy sessions every two weeks, had controlled her symptoms to the point that her psychiatrist felt confident Kathy was up to her East Coast adventure. Dr. Dorothy had written in her medical notes "go with my blessing," "find a good psychiatrist," "keep up with drug maintenance therapy."

Restricted to St. Mary's medical unit, Kathy received piece-meal care for her manic state. Short of the last several days of her hospital stay, she required the expensive and constant care of a bedside so-called specials nurse. Initially, restraints were used liberally because few of the specials nurses had adequate psychiatric training to know the techniques for talking a patient down. As well, Kathy was considered a danger to herself, and the low dose of Zyprexa was minimally effective in controlling symptoms.

Though Dr. Bob encouraged Dr. Jerome to aggressively adjust the medication, Dr. Jerome did not feel comfortable with that type of judgment call, and Dr. Bob was not around enough to monitor and correct dosage. As determined by behavioral health managed care policy, reimbursement for treatment in a nonnetwork hospital was far less than the value of Dr. Bob's time and effort. Consequently, his visits to Kathy were occasional. These virtually donated visits, however, were the interventions that brought Kathy's medical and psychiatric conditions under control.

Kathy was discharged 42 days after being admitted through the emergency room. Most of her symptoms of lithium toxicity resolved, though she still had slightly slurred speech. Dr. Bob called the psychiatrist in Grand Forks to confirm Kathy's history and the treatments that had been tried. He concluded that lithium and Effexor would be retained as the best way to control Kathy's bipolar disorder even with renal insufficiency. Before her discharge, he put Kathy on much lower doses and planned to follow her blood levels closely.

Dr. Jerome would follow Kathy's medical situation. Because he and Dr. Bob worked in separate noncommunicating clinical systems, they only could hope for smooth collaboration. Because of the exclusion rider for her kidney disease and out-of-network treatment for her behavioral health issues, when Kathy walked out of the hospital her portion of the bill was $52,000. Her retirement nest egg was severely reduced, with medical bankruptcy in the cards. Her name appearing on the roster of a public program was not inconceivable. Though her children and best friends lived in Grand Forks and could benefit her fragile health, she most likely would not be able to get insurance in North Dakota at this point. Her soiled medical records at best would qualify her for a high-risk policy at a premium rate that would bury her financially. Because her Blues health savings plan would not transfer to North Dakota, she was tied to Virginia with less than reliable coping skills.

If the U.S. health care environment required universal participation and portability of insurance as sketched out earlier in this chapter, there would have been no need for Kathy to hide the truth of her behavioral health service use or pay such high insurance rates. Her North Dakota policy would have made the move to Virginia with her. Because risk pools in systems with universal participation are based on the national population, Kathy's preexisting polycystic kidney disease would not have been excluded in the health package. By using illness severity groupers, such as the Johns Hopkins Adjusted Clinical Groups (ACGs) Case-Mix System, it would have been factored into the acuity level for the Blues in Virginia with a fair share of funds collected and earmarked for health management for all subscribers.

Unfortunately, this practical and equitable design was not available to Kathy. She was instead ensnared in a twisted net of bureaucracy. A long and grueling period of holding on telephone lines, writing letters, and requesting health record documentation in an effort to resolve the confusion of who owes what to whom will follow Kathy's hospital discharge. She likely will get lost on the waiting lists for disease or case management. Lawyers will join the fray. Her novel will not get written, and her health will deteriorate under the pressure. The irony in this bleak picture is that Kathy did not receive optimum care for the bipolar illness that complicated her medical illness, yet it was that very same treatment that threatened her financial good standing.

Kathy's situation appears to be the result of a confluence of unfortunate and rare circumstances, but it occurs commonly and in many forms in our system. Patients with concurrent illness like Kathy's account for one-fifth to one-third of total health care dollars spent. Ultimately, this patient group is forced to move to public programs and will use more services than do patients who have sufficient resources to buy insurance. Bad enough is that Kathy had to deal with two debilitating illnesses. Worse yet is that she was saddled with the challenge of getting treatment in a two-part system that has chosen to divorce the health of the body from the health of the mind.

There are big-system general medical issues that obviously come into play as we enter the analysis of Kathy's health needs, coverage, and service use. Insurance and coordinated care factors relating to her bumpy ride are important components in the discussion. It is a messy disjointed jam, so buckle your seat belts.

PURCHASING PHYSICAL AND BEHAVIORAL
HEALTH CARE

When Kathy moved to Virginia, she became her own health plan purchaser, whereas in North Dakota her employer provided it for her, and she played the system as well as the system played her. Recognizing the impact that psychiatric illness has on insurability, she hid her mental health treatment and eradicated the paper trail by paying cash. The special payment arrangement she made with Dr. Dorothy and the low cost of the medication prescribed for her made concealment possible. Because Kathy understood bipolar disorder was a disease just like a stomach ulcer or pneumonia, her drive to keep her mental health issues under wraps was not motivated by embarrassment. Rather, it was a stealth method by which she could avoid financial impediments that a stigmatized system had imposed on her. Regrettably, the charade also kept her lithium use for bipolar disorder a secret that ultimately imperiled her life.

Kathy's incentive for health coverage once she arrived in Virginia was different from the real estate agency through which she had previously been insured. Best Buy Realty looked on behavioral health care as a waste of money and went out of its way to find the most confining behavioral health benefits for its employees. It was not difficult to do so through an independent carved-out managed behavioral health company. The subcontracted behavioral health policy they purchased for their employees offered no substance-use disorder treatment options and no in-network mental health practitioners in the Grand Forks area other than several low-paid counselors who saw patients in crisis.

Whenever patients needed access to network psychiatrists, rigorous review procedures ensured that every dollar was spent for necessary care, waiting times were long, and the distance to the closest provider was in Fargo, 80 miles away. North Dakota was a nonparity state where disparate medical and behavioral health benefit restrictions were legal, thus co-pays were 50 percent of clinic charges for psychiatric services rather than the 20 percent assigned for general medical co-pays. Annual and lifetime limits for days of treatment, the number of clinic visits, and reimbursement rates for behavioral health providers also were adjusted downward in an effort to conserve health care dollars.

Because Virginia recently had passed parity legislation, Kathy anticipated a reduction in the financial and clinical discrimination she experienced in North Dakota when she tried to get her depression treated in the mental health sector. To her dismay, there were few differences between North Dakota and Virginia. Even though she had deceptively chosen to report only mild depression on her application to avoid a higher premium, she encountered a massive increase in the premium and a reduction in coverage for a simple Effexor prescription.

The HSA, presented as her only affordable option, had similar general medical and behavioral health cost and coverage inequities as did her North Dakota plan. The behavioral health provider network was significantly limited and accessed through a separate Web site from other practitioners serving Blues patients. Clinicians in general medicine and psychiatry practiced in independent locations, including hospitals. They had separate documentation systems and received payment through an independent coding and reimbursement process. Importantly, as Kathy later found out, there was also little communication between medical and behavioral health specialists even though they were presumably a part of the same system.

HEALTH PLAN MANAGEMENT OF PHYSICAL AND BEHAVIORAL HEALTH CARE

Kathy's health plan in North Dakota, Swift Care, had only 30,000 members served by local providers. It specialized in serving the needs of small companies, like Kathy's real estate firm. The contracts offered to the real estate firm's employees were bare bones because Best Buy Realty was trying to adjust to escalating medical inflation yet retain employer-based coverage.

Swift Care's utilization management efficiently and aggressively reviewed health service requests, medication, and medical device purchases for medical necessity. To support behavioral health services, Swift Care subcontracted with the independently owned managed behavioral health organization, Behavioral Value Distributors (BVD). Both managed the same Best Buy Realty employees using parallel, but often very different, processes.

- Each maintained its own sales and service personnel.
- Each wrote its own contract benefit descriptions.
- Each managed its own provider networks.
- Each processed (adjudicated) its own claims.
- Each performed its own utilization management.
- Each developed its own contract costs based on actuarial analysis from its own independent and discipline-specific data warehouses.
- Each paid claims from its own funding pools.
- Each executed its own quality-assurance programs.

Operating from two different internal data sets, there was no communication on any level between the medical and behavioral health services. This communication barricade between clinicians contributed to Kathy's ultimate health crisis, but other factors cannot be overlooked.

Had Kathy chosen to use her BVD benefit package to cover her mental health needs, at least her lithium prescriptions from Dr. Dorothy would have been on record. Determined to hide her bipolar condition to protect her future insurability, Kathy justified paying cash for psychiatric services by rationalizing that BVD's 50 percent co-pay requirement was nearly equal to what Dr. Dorothy charged her directly for private consultations. By so doing, she kept secret vital information that would have derailed the oncoming train. If Kathy's Grand Forks internist had known she was taking lithium, he would have been more compulsive about kidney testing. Likewise, Dr. Dorothy would have been more cautious about prescribing lithium had she been aware of Kathy's history of polycystic kidney disease.

While insuring Kathy, Best Buy Realty ostensibly accomplished what it set out to do. It minimized the cost of health care for its employees by separating general medical from behavioral health benefits but did so with little total health care savings and at the expense of Kathy's health and economic viability. Relying on Swift Care to cover most of her complaints while concealing the underlying behavioral element, Kathy used nearly 50 percent more general medical services than other employees. Because she never tapped into her behavioral health coverage, Best Buy Realty erroneously thought they had come out the winner. BVD did not raise its premium rate. A more thorough evaluation, however, would have revealed Swift Care's latest premium spike was to some extent attributable to Kathy's masking her behavioral complaints in order to take advantage of the better benefits offered in her medical package.

Arriving in Irvington, Kathy had hoped to narrow the gap and improve communication and coordination of her general medical and behavioral health care by going with a nationally recognized insurance company. But was she in better hands with the Blues? They managed their own behavioral health services, carved it in as opposed to carving it out like Swift Care had. Technically, they had one bottom line. Nonetheless, behavioral health was considered a different animal than physical health and managed the same as if it were carved out, like Swift Care and BVD. Medical and behavioral services, though owned by the Blues, each had its own administrative structure, provider networks, work flows, and budget. The only difference in Kathy's Blues coverage was that it cost her more.

To assume that many uninformed company health plan purchasers believe they are saving health care dollars by carving out behavioral health services is a safe bet. It is also safe to assume that many other patients on Kathy's disasterous path are hiding mental health illnesses to outsmart a system that plays favorites by carving out behavioral health care.

The unfortunate reality is that today millions of Kathys have a concealed interacting combination of general medical and psychiatric difficulties, many of whom can not get insurance even if they could afford the high premium. No matter if they were open books, listing every medication prescribed, and adhering religiously to every treatment, fund distributors hesitate to insure them. Failing to recognize the connection of quality care to lower costs, the health care system as a whole does not offer, nor does it champion, coordinated care for people with combined physical and mental illness even though higher service use and poor resolution rates are predictable outcomes.

Care Management

The purchasers of health care plans for large companies and corporations are as frugal as the fund distributors who sell the plans. Human resources (HR) personnel contracting for health and disability insurance for employees of these corporations are tireless in their attempts to staunch the outpouring of health dollars. Because complex and/or high-cost chronic general medical patients use a lion's share of the resources, many purchase managers request that health plan administrators, such as the Blues, provide case and disease management services to help them minimize health care consumption.

One of the more costly roadblocks in distributing the right care at the right time is the problem employees have in comprehending the complexity of the system. To avoid the hassles of deciphering industry jargon, locating a preferred provider, or wading through the paperwork of medical necessity permission slips many chronically ill patients make a beeline to an emergency room somewhere close to home. Using sick days or applying for disability is oftentimes easier than seeking help or following a treatment regime. In short, conserving the health care dollar is not a priority for the majority of this high-use group, but the employer outcry is loud and unanimous.

In response, the Blues and other major health plans have activated personalized telephone assistance programs, including disease and case management, employee assistance programs, health coaching, nurse lines, and disability management opportunities for patients with chronic/complex conditions. In fact, a great many health plans, whether for commercial, government, or individual clients, now include some type of assistance program, especially for complex and high-cost members. By the time Kathy was discharged from the hospital, she might have been considered a candidate for disease management, except that neither the excluded renal insufficiency nor the bipolar illness was among the diseases covered by the Blues disease management vendor in her plan.

Furthermore, even with a medical bill of $52,000 and obviously complex illness, she will not be near enough to the top of the list to qualify for the high-end case management health plan service. In reining in their administrative costs, of which case managers are a component, the Blues had substantially reduced its number of case managers. The maximum number they can assist per year is a mere 0.2 percent of their members, and Kathy would not make the cut.

INTEGRATED PHYSICAL AND BEHAVIORAL HEALTH CARE DELIVERY

To protect herself from the financial ravages of a catastrophic health problem, Kathy had insured herself (or thought she had). She took preventive measures to maintain her health. She trusted her doctors. So what happened?

Facing a life-threatening condition, Kathy was hospitalized for more than a month as a result of renal impairment complicated by a manic episode. Though her polycystic kidney disease was not covered by her health plan, her depression was. Because treatment for the depression was provided in a medical setting and outside of Kathy's behavioral health network, however, the health plan reimbursement rules did not apply. Even though the Blues owned the behavioral health contract covering Kathy's mental health, her mental health treatment fell outside the jurisdiction acceptable by them—a phenomenon not novel to a Kathy-type scenario.

The division of general medical and behavioral health services conspired against Kathy long before her adventure culminated in the Virginia fiasco. Kathy's North Dakota general internist, Dr. Karl, annually ordered routine preventive medical screens but had not monitored her kidney function because of her initial physical examination and normal laboratory findings five years earlier. Though he did know that she had bouts with depression from time to time, he was not aware that she was taking lithium. He also had taken pains not to mention the diagnosis of depression in his records even though he prescribed her Effexor.

Forced by reduced health plan reimbursements rates, Dr. Karl had to schedule more patients in order to meet his clinic administrator's financial expectations, which left him little time to establish doctor-patient relationships. Whether by reason of time constraints or not wanting to pry into Kathy's personal space, Dr. Karl did not take responsibility for her depression or its treatment. According to Dr. Sidney Wolfe, director of Public Citizen Health Research Group, "bad reactions to prescription drugs cause one and a half million hospital visits a year and about a hundred thousand deaths."[12] Yet despite this, Dr. Karl failed to inquire about Kathy's medication routines when she asked him to refill her Effexor prescription so she could use her medical benefits to pay for it. For this oversight, there would be severe consequences.

When Kathy began to experience dangerous mood swings, she recognized the symptoms as bipolar. The disease ran in her family, and well-versed in how to hide psychiatric treatment to protect her insurability, she took great pains to keep her visits with Dr. Dorothy and the subsequent lithium prescription off her medical records. Dr. Dorothy assisted many patients in similar situations and respected Kathy's wish for confidentiality. As part of that process, she never requisitioned Dr. Karl's records related to Kathy's medical conditions. If she had been apprised of Kathy's history of polycystic kidneys, she likely would have followed Kathy's kidney function more closely because of well-known lithium effects on the kidneys.

In Virginia, Kathy connected with Lynn, the nurse practitioner, for a routine annual exam. Loyal to old habits, Kathy omitted her psychiatric history and its treatment. The omission established the first link in a chain of events that would terminate in a long and expensive ordeal. Had Lynn taken the time to get the facts about Kathy's depression treatment, the water pill prescription to bring down Kathy's blood pressure probably would not have been written, especially the type of water pill Lynn gave Kathy because it is known to retard the elimination of lithium. Though Lynn tried to correct her inadvertent error, it was not soon enough. By the time she had collected and pieced together important medical facts, the second link was already in place. Dehydration, combined with the water pill on a hot summer day, had elevated the lithium level well into the toxic range. Kathy went to the hospital.

Kathy's hospital stay was complicated and prolonged, but not because lithium toxicity is difficult to treat, even in someone with poor kidney function. Yes, she required dialysis to flush the lithium as quickly as possible, but that is a bread-and-butter activity on any medical unit. Within a week, perhaps sooner, Kathy would have been out of the hospital had she not become manic during the course of her dialysis treatment.

The sudden withdrawal of the medications controlling Kathy's bipolar illness compounded what would have been a simple solution. Her unexpected manic behavior prevented the last dialysis treatment, and valuable time was lost because she was hospitalized in a medical setting that was ill-equipped and ill-staffed to handle psychiatric disorders. To further clutter the chaos, she was in a medical facility outside the network of her behavioral health contract and too medically unstable to be discharged and readmitted to an in-network psychiatric facility.

Dr. Jerome, Kathy's attending medical physician, administered the medications that the psychiatrist, Dr. Bob, advised. Untrained in the use of antimanic medications, however, he did not feel confident in treating Kathy aggressively enough to bring her mania rapidly under control. Dr. Bob was not a network provider in St. Mary's and, therefore, was available only sporadically. Electroconvulsive therapy, a quick and effective treatment for mania, was not available at St. Mary's, but Kathy could not be moved to Methodist Hospital, where such treatments were available, because their psychiatric unit would not assume the responsibility because of her kidney disease.

Finally, once Kathy's behavior was under control, it was a challenge to get her on a medication that would maintain her mood stability in the face of impaired kidney function, especially because many medications used to control bipolar illness are eliminated through the kidneys. This would require coordinated treatment by Dr. Jerome and Dr. Bob who had developed rapport during Kathy's hospital stay. Because they were physicians in separate networks, their efforts would be impeded by the system through which Kathy's treatment was supported.

Kathy's story is just one of thousands that can be told about the interaction of general medical and psychiatric illness operating in a two-part system. Putting her health in jeopardy, Kathy had to play games with her health plans and with the clinicians who treated her in order to get care for her psychiatric condition. Substantial challenges now await her, both clinically, in getting the coordination of general medical and psychiatric services that she needs, and economically, in maintaining financial solvency while trying to retain health insurance that will allow her to address her health issues.

Chapter 5

HOMEWORK

An idea is not worth much until a man is found who has the energy
and the ability to make it work.

—Anonymous

Kathy's type of clinical situation is common, very costly, and occurs at every
level in our health care system. To continue to deny these patients good care or
limit their access to treatment is not going to make them go away. Consuming
25 percent to 50 percent of the health care dollar, complex patients suffering with
psychiatric illness face enormous challenges, and without appropriate and timely
care, their numbers will continue to swell. Policy makers and critics alike agree
the separated system is riddled with inefficiencies, waste, poor management,
smothering costs, and inequitable coverage, but the machine grinds on, propagat-
ing more of the same.

Purchasers continue to buy the ineffective cost/quality health care packages
for their employees and members because that is what health plans offer. Providers and facilities persevere with separate treatment environments because health
plan reimbursement policies dictate it. Health plan administrators perpetuate general medical and behavioral health separation not because their customers are
satisfied, and maybe not even because they are convinced it works, but because it
makes them money!

Being aware of a problem is a step toward correcting it, and certainly few are
unaware of the problematic bureaucracy of the U.S. health care system. To effect
quality health care for the citizens of the United States, however, we need mavericks with a vision and the tenacity to dismantle and rebuild important components
of a failed system. To illustrate how positive change can occur, in this and the next

three chapters Alex, Edward, and Vicki are the mavericks who will set the wheels in motion.

* * *

Alex walked out of the executive staff board meeting after presenting the annual health-usage data for ECI, a major electronic medical records company now in its 15th year. He returned the notebook computer with the slide presentation into its port and watched a spring snowstorm swirl outside his office window. He felt lousy. In the last three years, health care costs had risen 13 percent, a 2 percent increase over his predecessor's poor record.

ECI's 5,000-strong workforce was predominantly healthy young professionals living in Denver where outdoor activities flourished year-round and health-conscious restaurants and groceries thrived. The company offered fresh salads, grilled chicken and salmon wraps, yogurt, fresh fruit, and vegetables in its cafeteria. It sponsored health club memberships and softball teams. Annually, the employee assistance program (EAP) promoted a weekend health fair for the employees and their families with access to cholesterol and blood sugar testing, bone density and lung capacity evaluations, and diet and exercise interventions for a nominal fee. Yet the health care cost challenge had not abated at ECI.

Part of the problem was that ECI was one of the subsidiaries of Telstar, an investment conglomerate owning 14 companies with a workforce of more than 60,000 employees and an additional 75,000 family members. Although ECI was perhaps the youngest and fastest growing of Telstar's holdings, the company also owned a number of larger, more mature operations with an older workforce in the Denver area. Though technically an employee of ECI, Alex had been hired with the understanding that he would be on the team that negotiated health plan contracts for all of Telstar because of his unique combination of medical and business backgrounds.

At the conclusion of Alex's presentation, an assembly of senior and associate officers had delivered their implied consensus loud and clear, "Get a handle on the costs or follow your predecessor out the door." With a doctorate in health care administration and 10 years' experience as a registered nurse on a general medical unit, Alex had felt confident taking the helm as Vice President of ECI's human resources (HR) division. He listened to the expectations and budget demands from the chain of command and kept current on all health plan products and modifications, the climate changes within the industry, and the employees' concerns.

Nevertheless, his boss clamored for cuts. The complaints on a recent health service satisfaction survey mounted. The Blues, Ecumenical Care, and Medical Mart, the three health plans with which ECI contracted for its employee benefit package, forecasted another 15 percent hike in next year's premiums, with neither provider service nor medication costs projected to level out. Months prior to the executive staff meeting, Alex saw the writing on the wall but could not find enough fat in his company benefit package to begin to know where to pare down.

Several years ago, he had changed from a fully insured product, in which the health plan took the financial risk for administrative and service claims costs, to a self-insured product that left the administrative costs with the health plan and shifted the claims costs to ECI. The switch gave ECI better control over decisions regarding benefit descriptions and service usage under the Employee Retirement Income Security Act (ERISA) laws. It also afforded the company more leverage in holding down costs. Taking advantage of the flexibility, Alex worked closely with the health plans to create benefit packages that required employees:

- To pay higher co-pays for more expensive providers, dependent on tier-based contracted discounts with the health plans.
- To preferentially choose generic over brand-name drugs and even mail-order medication from Canada when possible.
- To move toward health savings accounts that would supposedly curb excessive and unnecessary service use.

The health plans with which ECI contracted were expected to provide aggressive utilization review procedures to deter frivolous health service use and high-cost medical equipment. Case management services were included in the three packages. Ecumenical Care used a claims-based predictive modeling program that identified patients at high risk for excessive future claims as a trigger for case management. The two others targeted patients whose health care use had generated high costs in the past. Finally, consistent with Alex's abiding interest in ensuring quality care, he had purchased a disease management package from AdvancedDM for all employees and their families who had, or might have, diabetes, heart disease, asthma, end-stage kidney disease, and several rare but high-cost illnesses.

At the bidding of Mr. Kishi, the Chief Executive Officer (CEO) of the company, Alex had paid particular attention to psychiatric services in contract negotiations. As the final lap of the interview process before hiring Alex, Mr. Kishi had invited him for drinks at a neighborhood bistro for a personal chat regarding the expected contents of an ECI health benefit package. Alex ordered a Boulder microbrew and Mr. Kishi sipped a house wine while he told his story.

His daughter Misaki had anorexia with bulimic features. Though Mr. Kishi had maximum benefits through his Blues plan, the hospital could not register his 5-foot 7-inch, 98-pound, dehydrated daughter for psychiatric care when he brought her, limp and exhausted, into the admissions office. The hospital's small eating disorder unit was full, and Misaki would have to be put on a waiting list. Even then, admission was iffy because the Blues would not guarantee payment unless she was considered suicidal.

The emergency staff doctor recommended that Misaki continue her outpatient treatment to "turn things around." Mr. Kishi knew better. Without constant supervision, Misaki would not adhere to a calorie-controlled diet and nonexercise program. Mr. and Mrs. Kishi both monitored her diet like they would an infant with the stomach flu, but Misaki continued to lose weight. Promising to go to the arranged outpatient therapies, Misaki would instead run laps at the local high school track. The occasional times they escorted her to a session, the therapy would be forgotten at her next urge to binge and vomit. They could not stalk her every waking moment.

Using his executive weight, Mr. Kishi had talked directly to the Blues CEO with the intent of forcing the plan to accommodate his daughter or he would find another insurer for his company. The Blues CEO talked with the utilization review medical director, who in turn talked with the emergency room physician, but even with the brass demanding Misaki be admitted, there just were not enough beds on the eating disorders unit. Major purchaser's daughter or not, she was going to have to wait in line.

Clinically dehydrated with a blood pressure of 80/60 and abnormal electrolytes, Misaki was finally admitted to the general medical unit by the family internist. Despite Dr. Evans's numerous phone calls to rustle up a psychiatrist, none appeared. On the fourth and last day of her stay, a nurse clinician representing psychiatry sympathized with the Kishis but did not have a solution. Every effort to find an available bed for a severely ill eating-disorder patient on a psychiatric unit within a 50-mile radius and even the specialty eating-disorders unit in Denver was futile. Colorado, like 23 other states, had a documented shortage of psychiatric beds.

"My daughter was dying, Alex, and I would have paid a king's ransom to get her help." In desperation, the Kishis had coerced the Blues to pay for transportation to and from a treatment center in Arizona.

When Misaki completed the program in Arizona a month later, Mr. Kishi concluded that she was better but not well. Upon discharge, the Arizona treatment center had coordinated care with Misaki's Colorado internist, Dr. Evans, but he was not an eating disorder specialist. He could monitor weight, dehydration, and electrolyte disturbances on a regular basis but generally did not synchronize his care with eating-disorders programs. Specialty services for anorexia were available in the Denver area, but Misaki had already burned a number of those bridges.

"The path to behavioral health care is a minefield of missed moments," Mr. Kishi said sliding his Visa card onto the tabletop. "Remember my story."

Alex had. In discussions with all of ECI's health plans and the vendors providing other health-enhancing services, he urged collaboration between general medical and behavioral care managers for patients with complex problems. He wanted to avoid duplication of services and complications due to lack of communication between providers. Ecumenical Care carved out its behavioral health to BVD, Medical Mart to Ferdinand Behavioral (FB). The Blues owned its own under the product name Blue Behavioral. All three rigorously claimed that they encouraged coordination of care between mental health/substance use and physical health providers.

To strengthen behavioral health coverage, Alex purchased a depression disease management package from FB for employees who also received assistance from AdvancedDM's disease managers covered by Medical Mart. Though a number of employee complaints made note of a lack of communication between AdvancedDM's and FB's disease managers in assessing an employee's coexisting conditions, the numbers suggested a significant pre- to postbehavioral health cost reduction for employees accessing both services, though not enough to significantly slash the company's overall health care costs.

Alex stared out the window, his thoughts ricocheting like pinballs. Old tapes played back from classrooms to health care seminars, think tanks to conferences—spending money on psychiatric care is like pouring it down a rat hole. He knew it was an all too familiar sentiment reflecting something deep within the psyche of a society that musters a prejudice against mental health and substance-use disorders and every other flavor of psychological difficulties—almost a universal primordial disgust. A cornucopia of negative inflection attends behavioral health terminology in which "Oh my god, she's so neurotic!" and "What a psycho!" are common put-downs uttered to identify insignificant everyday personality glitches.

"Get a grip!" and "Get over it!" are standard pep talks given out freely to friends or family who suffer unrequited love or manic depression, substance-use disorders or a broken fingernail. For many hearty-stock Americans, that is enough to jump-start a positive change, but to the chronically ill or severely addicted, it is a bad joke. Anyone working a 12-step recovery program knows the devil never sleeps. A rescued schizophrenic given an apartment, a job, new clothes, and balanced meals likely will escape back to the streets within months, panhandling for spare change and smoking cigarette butts retrieved from city trash receptacles unless he remains in treatment. A cheering section, though noble, will not make a dent in his prognosis.

From his nursing experience, Alex knew that one of the worst impediments about having a mental disorder was the shame. The implied snicker discouraged many from seeking the help they needed, though at any given time, an estimated 1 in 10 employees experience mental misfires that cost companies billions of dollars in lost productivity and absenteeism.[1] Alex did not kid himself that millions of employees nationwide, probably hundreds at ECI alone, were hiding mental dysfunction under the guise of medical problems to protect their careers. A 2004 study reported that 41 percent of employees with depression felt they could not acknowledge their illness without jeopardizing career upward mobility in the company, and that they definitely did not get a fair shake in health care benefits.[2]

Ten years on a general medical unit gave Alex a broad sense of the foibles of managed medical health care, and he never could understand the rationale behind moving psychiatric treatment to an independently managed sector. He often had wondered if there was a connection between scaling back on mental health and substance-use disorder coverage and increased health costs down the line. Or was conventional wisdom right? Money for psychiatric care was money wasted. The concept was certainly strong at Telstar. He had been outvoted for the past three years by the others on the negotiating team. Telstar retained higher co-pays and annual and lifetime spending limits for behavioral health in their contracts.

If the corporate office demanded leaner health care budgets, most chief health plan negotiators did not think twice about tightening benefits for mental health and substance-use disorders. After all it was not "real" disease. According to an annual benefits survey conducted by the Society for Human Resource Management, the percentage of employers offering mental health benefits has tapered off from 84 percent to 76 percent in an effort to reduce health care costs.[3]

No doubt, directing the hit at behavioral health would be the simple solution, but Alex contemplated the stakes. He remembered meeting Misaki Kishi, watching her fragile body lunge at the volleyball net at the company picnic. He remembered the statistics on common changes in workplace behavior when mental dysfunction interfered, the frequent sick days, irritability, missed deadlines, avoidance of crucial decisions, and forgotten directives. And he remembered the human resource department's analysis of the behavioral health-related complaints logged by ECI employees. It was not pretty.

He swiveled toward his computer, put on his glasses, and brought up the complaint file summary from both employees and their clinicians.

- Insurance pays more readily for treatment of an illness with a medical diagnosis than a psychological diagnosis (employee).
- Impersonal 800 numbers to access health service for psychiatric matters (employee and physical health clinician).
- Limited list of available in-network providers for counseling on mental health and substance-use disorder issues and long distances to travel to get to an in-network psychiatrist accepting patients (employees and physical health clinicians).
- Long waiting periods for first appointments, especially with psychiatrists and child psychiatrists (employees and physical health clinicians).
- Denials for inpatient and/or outpatient care based on "no medical necessity" or "exceeded benefit limits" when nothing else is available (employees).
- Primary and specialty medical care physicians give poor mental health care and follow-up, yet they do not make referrals for emotional problems due to benefit restrictions or just to avoid hassles (mental health clinician).
- Infighting between physical and behavioral health coinsurers about who pays for clinical services when both physical and behavioral care are needed and given (employee).
- Scarcity of reasonably spaced psychiatric follow-up appointments (employee and family member).
- Frustration with current therapist, but no alternatives available (employee).
- Hassles of seeing two providers in different locations and on different days because of payment restrictions to address co-occurring medical and psychiatric illnesses (employee, family, physical and mental health doctors located in the same clinic).
- Lack of communication between mental health specialists and primary care physicians (employees).

Obviously, the majority of complaints zeroed in on limited access to mental health and substance-use care and the hoops employees or their family members had to jump through to get an appointment with a psychiatrist or other mental health and substance-use disorder clinician, if they could get an appointment at all. Delays in getting in for treatment were a special concern, especially in dire situations—a suicidal child or a husband toting a gun to work inside his brief case. It was not necessarily that they could not get seen in an emergency. There was always the emergency room. It was the aftercare that was the problem.

They were all valid complaints. Alex was well aware of the industry's rejection of the remarkable interrelationship of the mind and body, but it went beyond his job description to change the viewpoint of an entire industry. He closed the file.

It was after five o'clock. But for an occasional beep and burp of a machine, the office was quiet. Alex turned on his notebook computer and pulled up his Power-Point presentation. Two particular consecutive slides had caught his attention at the executive meeting, slides he had authored and edited but during the presentation he had seen from a fresh perspective. He clicked the advance key. The percentage of the total health care dollar spent on behavioral health had dropped from 4.1 percent to 3.4 percent over the last three years, yet antidepressants were now at the top of the chart as the most frequently prescribed medication for Telstar's 60,000 employees and 75,000 family members (Figure 5.1; although many of the figures, tables, and cost/usage calculations in the text in this and following chapters are simulations for the fictitious company, ECI, the health plans that it works with, and the Providence Hospital system, they reflect real numbers from real employers, health plans, and health care delivery systems with similar characteristics to those found in Chapter 5 through Chapter 8), of which 9 percent were from ECI. Because ECI's individual statistics closely paralleled those of Telstar employees who had identical coverage, Alex had felt comfortable in using the larger Telstar data set for a good portion of his presentation at the board meeting.

He clicked to the next slide. The cost drivers were not isolated to serious heart disease, diabetes, or cancer patients, but rather to patients falling into the broad category of behavioral health (Figure 5.2). Clicking the two slides back and forth,

Figure 5.1 Annual cost of top 10 drug groups.
A review of Telstar claims information shows that antidepressants were at the top of the list of most costly medications for the 135,000 employees and dependents in 2004. They accounted for nearly $9 million in prescription medications annually.

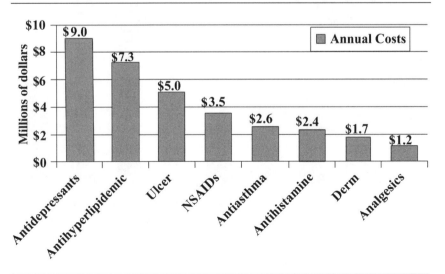

he studied the numbers and wondered what truth lay buried in the discrepancy? Before he took the ax to behavioral health, he intended to find out.

Nearly a foot of snow had fallen by the time Alex left his office that evening. The salt trucks were out, cross-country skiers glided down side streets, and street lamps glinted on the powder drifts. He arched his back and breathed in the sharp air. He had a path to follow and welcomed the quest.

PSYCHIATRIC CARE TODAY

Determined to find a way to ensure good health care for the ECI employees and their families and to keep the company strong, Alex spent the next five months looking for answers to three specific questions.

1. Can patients like Misaki get good health care when mental health and substance-use disorder care is handled independently from physical health?

2. How do mental health and substance-use disorders impact productivity and disability costs?

3. What are the merits of integrating physical health with mental health/substance-use disorder care?

Here is what Alex found.

Figure 5.2 Comparative trends in total annual costs of health care for Telstar employees with selected illnesses.
When compared to diabetes, cancer, and heart disease treatment, behavioral health care contributed almost twice as much as each to health care spending for Telstar employees. It also was rising at a more rapid rate from year to year.

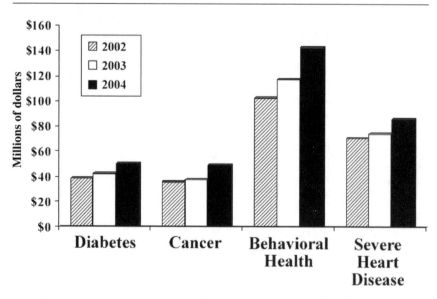

Question 1: Treatment of Mental Health and Substance-Use Disorders

Prevalence studies of psychiatric illness date back to the early 1970s and have been replicated several times at intervals through the years. The latest study in 2004 confirmed that two-thirds of patients, consistently and over time, received *no* treatment for their mental health and substance-use disorders (Figure 5.3).[4] The reasons are varied, but most frequently noted is that patients with psychiatric difficulties do not advocate well for themselves, nor do they know how to get help if, in fact, they know they need it.

Applying this statistic to Telstar, Alex recognized that behavioral health complaint files probably did not then accurately represent the number of employees with mental health and substance-use disorders. The studies indicated that of the 30 percent who did receive treatment, two-thirds sought treatment from

Figure 5.3 Two-thirds of patients with mental illness receive no treatment. Epidemiological studies since the early 1990s consistently show that two-thirds of people with mental health and substance-use disorder problems receive no treatment at all. For the third who do, most treatment is given by clinicians in the physical health sector who have limited mental health training and virtually no access to mental health and substance-use disorder professional support.

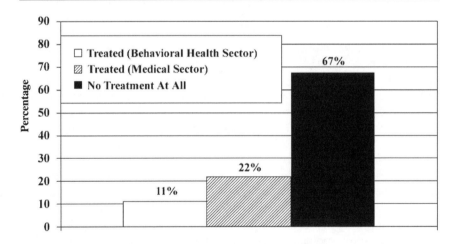

Source: Adapted from W. E. Narrow, D. S. Rae, L. N. Robins, D. A. Regier, "Revised Prevalence Estimates of Mental Disorders in the United States," *Archives of General Psychiatry* 59 (2002): 115–23; K. Demyttenaere, R. Bruffaerts, J. Posada-Villa, I. Gasquet, V. Kovess, J. P. Lepine, M. C. Angermeyer, S. Bernert, G. de Girolamo, P. Morosini, et al., "Prevalence, Severity, and Unmet Need for Treatment of Mental Disorders in the World Health Organization World Mental Health Surveys," *Journal of the American Medical Association* 291, no. 21 (2004): 2581–90; R. C. Kessler, O. Demler, R. G. Frank, M. Olfson, H. A. Pincus, E. E. Walters, P. Wang, K. B. Wells, and A. M. Zaslavsky, "Prevalence and Treatment of Mental Disorders, 1990 to 2003," *New England Journal of Medicine* 352, no. 24 (2005): 2515–23; R. C. Kessler, W. T. Chiu, O. Demler, K. R. Merikangas, and E. E. Walters, "Prevalence, Severity, and Comorbidity of 12-Month *DSM-IV* Disorders in the National Comorbidity Survey Replication," *Archives of General Psychiatry* 62, no. 6 (2005): 617–27.

Table 5.1
Most Telstar Employee Psychiatric Medication Prescriptions Are Written by Nonpsychiatrists

Psychiatrists prescribe
    26% of all psychiatric medications
    19% of psychiatric medications for discrete employees

Nonpsychiatrists prescribe
    74% of all psychiatric medications
    81% of psychiatric medications for discrete employees

Note: According to pharmacy records.

their primary or medical specialty care physicians. This was confirmed by Telstar's internal prescription data showing that nonpsychiatrists (Table 5.1) wrote the majority of psychiatric medication prescriptions.

Alex knew all too well that few general medical doctors were comfortable treating psychiatric illnesses. They told him so. They had not been trained to diagnose or treat psychiatric conditions, nor did they feel that they had the time with all their patients' other physical illnesses. Alex heard that many general internists and family physicians willingly would refer patients to a psychiatrist or psychologist if they could locate one without a three-month wait, let alone one that was in their patient's health plan network. It was just easier for them to write a prescription and see the patient again in a month or two and hope for the best. Psychotherapy was rarely considered because it was like sending their patients into a black box.

Although general practitioners had the best interests of their patients at heart, when they tried to treat mental health problems in their patients (more than 90 percent with medication) without behavioral health specialist assistance, numerous studies showed that symptom improvement was unlikely to occur.[5] It was only when primary care physicians worked with case managers in their clinics who were savvy about mental health and substance-use disorders, had time to develop a good relationship with the patient, and followed adherence and outcomes that treatment success occurred.

In clinical practice, this, of course, was not possible. Mental health and substance-use disorder practitioners, including case managers, received insufficient reimbursement for the services they provided to work in primary care clinics. Few internists or family practice physicians were willing to subsidize mental health support from their own earnings. Misaki's internist, Dr. Evans, is a case in point. He did not have access to a mental health specialist in his clinic, could not get Misaki into a psychiatric unit, and could not identify a follow-up program even though Misaki had serious psychiatric illness.

Alex also was aware that a lot of hide-and-seek games went on in the interest of getting paid for treatment time spent by primary care doctors. They nearly always miscoded depression and anxiety as headache, back pain, dizziness, or some other convenient somatic symptom to make sure that they got paid and that patients did not get tagged with a psychiatric label.[6] Patients also came out ahead if they opted for treatment on the medical side. Their co-pays were

20 percent of billed charges instead of 50 percent, the standard for mental health and substance-use disorder visits in Telstar's contracts. Furthermore, employees did not have to use their limited number of allocated annual behavioral health visits when they saw their primary care physician for psychiatric treatment. In the event that more specialized care was needed, they would still have mental health and substance-use disorder service access remaining. Little did they know that the treatment they received was unlikely to alter their illness.

Unlike for physical health and mental health/substance-use disorder services, all prescription medications, psychiatric or not, are paid from one pool of money; therefore, patients can get prescriptions for depression and anxiety from their primary care doctor. Doing so is easy, less expensive, and the most face-saving way to get treatment. It is, however, by no means the quickest or least expensive route to recovery, as Alex was coming to realize.

Furthermore, in the primary care setting, there is a solid relationship between the number of somatic symptoms that a patient has and coexisting anxiety or depression (Figure 5.4).[7] Most often, patients who were seen for their numerous somatic

Figure 5.4 The number of unexplained somatic symptoms predicts the presence of mood and anxiety disorders.
Nearly a decade ago, Kroenke and colleagues showed that the number of unexplained physical complaints was closely associated with the presence of depression and anxiety.

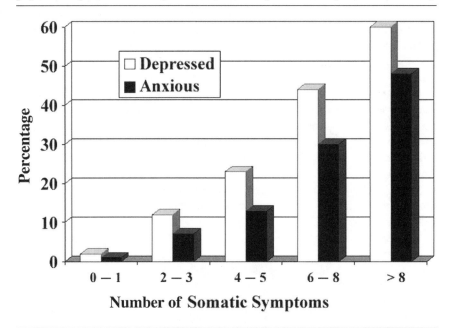

Number of Somatic Symptoms

Source: Adapted from K. Kroenke, R. L. Spitzer, J. B. Williams, M. Linzer, S. R. Hahn, F. V. deGruy, III, and D. Brody, "Physical Symptoms in Primary Care: Predictors of Psychiatric Disorders and Functional Impairment," *Archives of Family Medicine* 3, no. 9(1994): 774–79.

complaints were labeled *treatment resistant,* or simply shunted into the demeaning category of "hypochondriac" and dismissed to assail the next general practitioner. A diagnosis and treatment for anxiety and/or depression were rarely given.

Half of all visits to primary care doctors, therefore, were a result of symptoms unexplained by a physical illness, such as chest pain, stomach bloating, and shortness of breath. Not surprisingly, these patients underwent unnecessary tests with insignificant findings, but not without significant health risk and expense. A $2,500 procedure to rule out a blocked artery is a gigantic bill when simple psychiatric screening, done early, would have uncovered panic disorder.

Substantial empirical data now recognized that the most common psychiatric conditions treated in a medical setting are related to anxieties, including illness worry, and depression. Translating this information to ECI readily cleared up the discrepancy that had inspired Alex's quest for answers. The majority of ECI employees and their family members were going to general medicine physicians to have their anxieties and depression ineffectively treated with either poor psychiatric medication prescribing habits or tests and medications for unexplained physical complaints. Total health care costs thus were on the upswing. Meanwhile, the independently measured mental health and substance-use disorder budget trended downward. Few of the many patients with psychiatric illness ever made it to the psychiatric setting. One of the puzzle pieces slid nicely into place: low spending on behavioral health services but huge spending on unnecessary physical health tests and treatments.

Particularly interesting to Alex were patients with chronic medical illnesses who ran an exceptionally high risk for concurrent psychiatric illness.[8] The inaccessibility to coordinated care literally exacerbated their illnesses. They become a fixed cost on health care rosters. Patients with diabetes, heart disease, back pain, and so forth with co-occurring depression regularly tallied up Herculean health costs as a study Alex found by Druss and colleagues predicted (Table 3.5).[9]

In recalling conversations with clinicians he had interviewed, Alex understood that poor outcomes from an interaction of physical and behavioral problems set up a breeding ground for complications. Tantamount to symptom reversal is treatment adherence, but often depressed or anxious people with complex/chronic illnesses have difficulty following diets, exercising, conducting home tests, such as finger stick sugar levels and blood pressures, and keeping doctor appointments or therapy sessions.[10] Without adequate intervention for anxiety and depression along with monitoring for physical health adherence to treatment, these patients did not get better.

It appeared to Alex that in an attempt to preserve the health care dollar, a table tennis game using a human Ping-Pong ball was standard procedure in dealing with difficult and complex patients. The attention of both managed care systems focused on process rather than outcome—on shifting costs rather than eliminating them. Right there in his own backyard, Misaki's situation clearly demonstrated to Alex the systematic exercise of penny-wise and pound-foolish.

Because mental health and substance-use disorder care in the Denver area had been cut to the bone, Misaki could not get good care until she was transported to an expensive facility in Arizona, a thousand miles away from home. Regrettably, the good care would be temporary and unsustainable back home in Denver without a major revamp of a desperately insufficient mental health care system.

During his research, Alex ran across an interesting assessment of the introduction of managed behavioral health business practices at a manufacturing company on the East Coast.[11] Several largely behavioral health plan–funded studies consistently showed that using strict utilization management techniques—*Do not approve payment for treatment unless it is absolutely medically necessary, especially if it is inpatient or costly*—would yield an approximate 40 percent savings from the behavioral health budget. The East Coast manufacturer purchased such a plan and then measured the impact. As managed behavioral health practices went online and for three years thereafter, it tracked the medical budget, the mental health and substance-use disorder budget, and employee absenteeism.

The investigators found that behavioral health costs decreased the predicted 38 percent but, at the same time, medical health costs increased 37 percent for the employees who used psychiatric services. A net increase in the annual cost of care amounted to $130 per employee who used health services in 1993 dollars (Figure 5.5). During the same period, there was a 33 percent greater number of days absent from work compared to employees who did not use behavioral health services.

Figure 5.5 Behavioral health carve-outs increase total annual health care cost.
Following the introduction of managed behavioral health business practices in a manufacturer's employees over three years, Rosenheck and colleagues were able to demonstrate that reported behavioral health savings merely shifted to physical health benefit payments with a net increase in annual cost per employee of $130 in 1993 dollars. Absenteeism also increased by 30 percent compared to those who used no mental health services during this time.

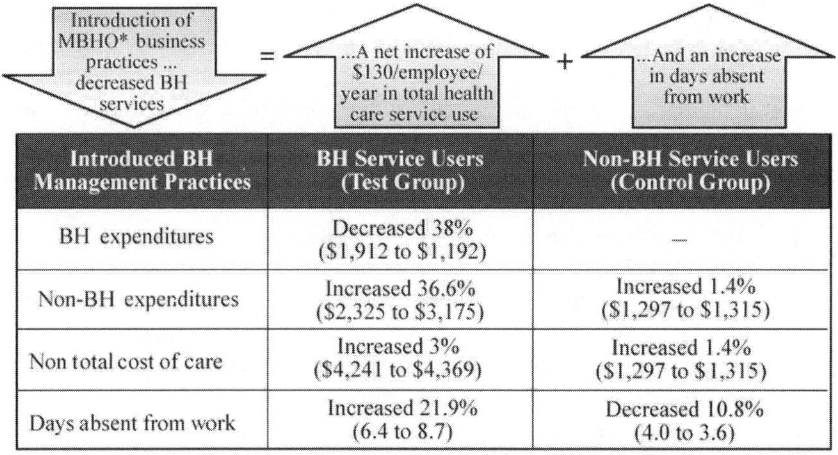

| Introduction of MBHO* business practices … decreased BH services | = | …A net increase of $130/employee/ year in total health care service use | + | …And an increase in days absent from work |

Introduced BH Management Practices	BH Service Users (Test Group)	Non-BH Service Users (Control Group)
BH expenditures	Decreased 38% ($1,912 to $1,192)	—
Non-BH expenditures	Increased 36.6% ($2,325 to $3,175)	Increased 1.4% ($1,297 to $1,315)
Non total cost of care	Increased 3% ($4,241 to $4,369)	Increased 1.4% ($1,297 to $1,315)
Days absent from work	Increased 21.9% (6.4 to 8.7)	Decreased 10.8% (4.0 to 3.6)

*Managed behavioral health organization

Source: Adapted from R. A. Rosenheck, B. Druss, M. Stolar, D. Leslie, and W. Sledge, "Effect of Declining Mental Health Service Use on Employees of a Large Corporation," *Health Affairs (Project Hope)* 18, no. 5 (1999): 193–203.

The association between increased health service use and reduced productivity in people accessing health service for mental health and substance-use issues is evident and certainly questions whether the techniques used to control behavioral health costs do not merely shift them from the psychiatric budget to the medical, with greater work impairment to boot. In this longitudinal study, the manufacturer spent more than $1 million more per year in health service usage by introducing managed behavioral health business practices into the company's health care package, a net loss that did not begin to calculate the cost of disability and lost employee productivity.

Question 2: Productivity and Disability

Alex did not have to go far to find out the impact of illness, both physical and psychiatric, on work productivity. Dr. Benjamin, an internist and psychiatrist, had been a longtime physician reviewer for the disability vendor ECI employed to process family leave and disability claims, Work Return, Inc. (WRI). For more than thirty years, Dr. Benjamin had served patients in his own brand of an integrated practice, and though nearing retirement, his dedication to helping employees find their way back to more productive lives after short- and long-term disabilities had not wavered.

Disability for psychiatric conditions constituted about 30 percent to 40 percent of claims, either as the primary problem or, more commonly, in association with a concurrent physical disability, such as low back pain, arthritis, heart disease, and the like.[12] Dr. Benjamin, familiar with the clinical and medical care cost impact that comorbid psychiatric illness had on an underlying physical condition, explained that high medical expenditures were small potatoes in terms of overall cost to companies.

With the rising costs of health care, six large corporations representing nearly 375,000 employees in 43 states convened to better understand the true total costs of ailing employees.[13] What they found, with the exception of heart disease and respiratory disorders, was that employees with concurrent medical and behavioral illnesses account for 50 percent to 90 percent of costs related to illness. These employees worked fewer hours, used more health care dollars, and were more likely to end up on short- and/or long-term disability (Table 5.2).

The whopping costs, however, were incurred not by medical costs or disability payments but as a result of diminished work capacity. Reviewing an isolated case, medical costs for a patient with chronic headaches, including migraines, were 8 percent of the total health care expenditure. Absences and/or short-term disability represented 3 percent, and 89 percent of the expense to the employer resulted from poor work functionality.

We all can relate to the effects of the common cold. Our energy is depleted and our focus out of whack. We feel lethargic and grumpy and want to go home, where we can crawl under a warm quilt and forget about it. *Presenteeism* is a relatively new term coined to describe this condition, and it is a source of concern to every

Table 5.2
Ten Health Conditions' Total Medical and Productivity Costs

	Medical	Absence/ Short-term Disability	Presenteeism	Total
Allergy	$29	$20	$222	$271
Arthritis	$46	$29	$252	$327
Asthma	$19	$9	$72	$100
Any cancer	$61	$7	$76	$144
Depression and mental illness	$54	$48	$246	$348
Diabetes	$75	$23	$159	$257
Heart disease	$266	$32	$71	$368
Hypertension	$91	$54	$247	$392
Migraine/headache	$17	$7	$189	$214
Respiratory disorders	$62	$39	$33	$134
Average	**$72**	**$26**	**$157**	**$255**

Note: Goetzel and colleagues showed that depression and mental health problems are second only to hypertension and heart disease as a health-related cost to employers. *Presenteeism,* the term used to describe employees who are at work but unproductive, accounts for nearly two-thirds of the cost of illness to employers.

Source: Adapted from R. Z. Goetzel, S. R. Long, R. J. Ozminkowski, K. Hawkins, S. Wang, and W. Lynch, "Health, Absence, Disability, and Presenteeism Cost Estimates of Certain Physical and Mental Health Conditions Affecting U.S. Employers," *Journal of Occupational and Environmental Medicine* 46, no. 4 (2004): 398–412.

HR department. The financial strength and viability of every company, large or small, depends on the vitality of its workforce.

As part of his participation at WRI, Dr. Benjamin focused not only on making sure that employees were getting and following through with their doctors' treatment programs, he also facilitated use of on-site resources to improve their health and work productivity. In coordination with EAPs, Dr. Benjamin worked with managers on how to recognize performance issues and help employees work through them.

It is not uncommon that an employee returning from disability leave will have a ripple effect on the rest of the employees. Employee conflicts arise or copycat symptoms occur in employees trying to protect themselves from excess workloads caused by their less productive colleagues. Without apparent reason, a once highly industrious department will mysteriously slip into slack production. With the assistance of the EAP team and disease management, health promotion (HP), and disability management when needed, Dr. Benjamin developed work reentry plans that allowed employees to ease back into a full schedule.

Responding to health care data noting that threefold to almost tenfold more employees accessed health services for psychiatric issues than they did for diabetes, cancer, or severe heart disease, such as that found in Telstar employees (Figure 5.6), Dr. Benjamin wasted no time in targeting that population. Perhaps the greatest challenge he faced in his role as physician-reviewer for WRI was arranging psychiatric treatment for employees with either primary psychiatric illness, such as depression, anxiety, substance-use disorder, and so forth, or secondary mental health or substance-use disorders related to an existing acute or chronic physical illness.

Dr. Benjamin also challenged general medical clinicians involved in treatment of employees or their family members to monitor behavioral health as compulsively as they did medical progress and to aggressively help them get better. One of the internists Dr. Benjamin contacted responded curtly, "I haven't performed a formal mental health examination on a patient since medical school, and now you are asking me to fill out a Physician Health Questionnaire [PHQ-9] documenting symptoms of depression! I don't think so."

Being a member of their guild, Dr. Benjamin helped internists come into compliance with his wishes. Those with whom he worked repeatedly became comfortable seeing their depressed patients more often while systematically recording symptom changes. If they felt overwhelmed, Dr. Benjamin encouraged them to get assistance from a psychiatrist. "Your patients' health depends on it."

The majority of employees that Dr. Benjamin worked with were routinely and ineffectively treated either solely by their primary care physician or by a primary care physician in combination with a non-outcome-oriented therapist. Originally, these unsuccessful cases came to Dr. Benjamin's attention six to eight weeks into the disability. Alert to the ramifications in both patient suffering and expense in high-risk employees, he urged WRI to use an initial provider support questionnaire that assessed clinical change prior to reinstating the employee to a full work schedule. By so doing, a measure of susceptibility of relapse and reasonable workload expectations could be defined.

From physicians and therapists, Dr. Benjamin expected clinical treatment and follow-up that would ensure the employee the best chance of improving and

Figure 5.6 Comparative annual number of 135,000 Telstar employees and dependents seeking help for high-cost conditions.
Part of the reason that costs were so high to Telstar for behavioral disorders was because they occurred in a much higher percentage of employees.

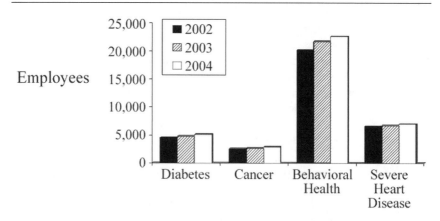

returning to work in a functional state. Often this included bringing in the assistance of a psychiatrist or a psychologist to get things back on track as well as the contributions of EAP and disease management programs. When psychotherapy appeared appropriate, this would be encouraged. Nearly always, follow-up contact would assess change.

After reviewing the gathered research on the symbiotic relationship of work productivity and behavioral health, Alex was well apprised of the direct and indirect costs of both physical and behavioral health. The extremely high costs associated with disability benefits, medical expenses for physical complaints without organic causes, and reduced work productivity trumped the cost of supporting and assuring outcome-oriented and coordinated mental health and substance-use disorder intervention.

Question 3: Effect of the Treatment of Behavioral Health Disorders

Alex had accumulated hard facts that behavioral health conditions occurred frequently and were being poorly managed, especially in the general medical sector in which the majority of treatment was given. Ineffectively treated mental health and substance-use disorders persisted and were associated with higher medical, pharmacy,

Figure 5.7 Annual claims expenditures for 250,000 patients with behavioral health service use are nearly doubled.
Total year-to-year health care costs for people with mental health and substance-use disorders have been shown by Kathol and colleagues to be twice the rate of those without mental health and substance-use disorders. The majority of service use in these individuals is for physical complaints and medications.

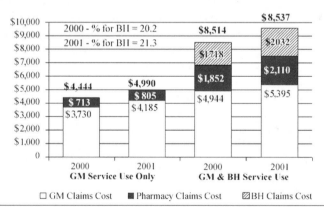

Percentage % of population: general medical (GM) service use: 74.9%; behavioral health (BH) service use: 10.0%; no service use: 15.1%

Source: R. G. Kathol, D. McAlpine, Y. Kishi, R. Spies, W. Meller, T. Bernhardt, S. Eisenberg, K. Folkert, and W. Gold, "General Medical and Pharmacy Claims Expenditures in Users of Behavioral Health Services," *Journal of General Internal Medicine* 20, no. 2 (2005): 160–67.

and productivity costs far in excess of the paltry 2 percent to 3 percent of the health dollar being devoted to psychiatric treatment. In fact, in the current system, nearly 70 percent of people with psychiatric disorders were receiving no treatment, and if they were, any behavioral health cost savings realized with carved-out management practices relied on shifting higher service usage to the physical health side (Figure 5.7).[14]

By limiting the use of a high number of unnecessary medications, tests, and referrals in those with unexplained somatic complaints and by assisting patients with chronic physical conditions to better adhere to their medical treatments, it was theoretically possible to lower the total cost of care when effective behavioral health interventions were given. Early studies failed to show this cost offset because the models of integration used were rudimentary and/or follow-up time for symptom improvement and then reduced health care use was insufficient. This trend, however, reversed.

By 2000, several integrated intervention models showed cost offset, mainly when 18- to 24-months follow-up was used to measure results. During the first six months after treatment initiation, costs actually increased, a reflection that psychiatric interventions were being given. Within a year, employees (patients) got back to their normal personal routines and workplace productivity. By this time, health use savings had now compensated for early treatment costs. Studies using outcome-changing models with 12-month follow-up were usually budget neutral. From 12 to 24 months, the real value kicked in. Symptoms resolved, health care costs went down, and family leave or disability days diminished in company records.

Targeted populations with illness characteristics that put them into frequent-user complex patient categories demonstrated improvement when behavioral health care practitioners and/or case managers worked alongside physical health caregivers. This was true for employees with depression, anxiety, substance abuse, and somatization seen in integrated clinics where physical and mental health/substance-use disorder clinicians work together in treating patients. It was also true for high-end users, meaning those admitted to general hospitals with serious medical illness who developed delirium, a debilitating and often lethal inpatient complication. Alex was impressed that integrated care models were available and that they worked. Unfortunately, few knew about them or used them.

A good example of how integrated care has an economic impact on general medical patients with concurrent physical and behavioral disorders, such as for an employee like Eva from Chapter 1, caught his eye. The results showed that patients who were depressed as well as diabetic and/or elderly (Figure 5.8) used nearly $1,000 less total health resources over two years when integrated practices were used.[15] Economic outcome changes were directly due to improvement of the clinical health of those exposed to integrated approaches to care. Although not measured, Alex reasoned this would translate into additional productivity and reduced disability.

Similar impressive results could be seen in patients with medical comorbidity and alcoholism. Integrating medical care with substance-use disorder treatment improved abstinence rates and reduced total cost (Table 5.3).[16] Based on this information, it made just as much sense to Alex to include substance-use disorder treatment in ECI's benefit package as diabetes or cardiac care. Although alcoholism is related to inability to control the intake of alcohol, diabetes and heart disease are

Figure 5.8 Integrating depression, diabetic, and geriatric care lowers biannual total health care costs.
Several research groups have demonstrated that coordinating physical and mental health treatment in diabetic and elderly patients with depression leads to better clinical outcomes and lower total health care costs. These improved outcomes appear to persist over time.

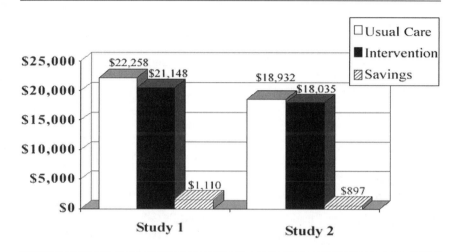

Source: Adapted from W. Katon, J. Unutzer, M.Y. Fan, J. W. Williams, Jr., M. Schoenbaum, E. H. Lin, and E. M. Hunkeler, "Cost-Effectiveness and Net Benefit of Enhanced Treatment of Depression for Older Adults with Diabetes and Depression," *Diabetes Care* 29, no. 2 (2006): 265–70; E.M. Hunkeler, W. Katon, L. Tang, J. W. Williams, Jr., K. Kroenke, E. H. Lin, L. H. Harpole, P. Arean, S. Levine, L. M. Grypma et al., "Long Term Outcomes from the IMPACT Randomised Trial for Depressed Elderly Patients in Primary Care," *British Medical Journal* 332, no. 7536 (2006): 259–63.

equally related to inability to control intake of food. If there are treatments that work for alcohol dependence that can get employees back to work and productive, it should be just as available as treatment of diabetes and heart disease.

* * *

At the fast approaching ECI executive meeting, Alex would be expected to show how he intended to bring down the rising health care costs. Because the success or failure of his presentation would mark a pivotal point in his career, he aimed to be thorough, all bases covered. To that end, he called the Telstar actuary to confirm the statistics that would constitute the basic premise for demanding a change in health care benefits and redirection of ECI's and, by inference, Telstar's health plans.

Alex had met Helen long ago when he was a registered nurse and she was working as a nurse's aide while completing her college degree in accounting. Though there was a 20-year gap in their music tastes, their careers had paralleled. Shortly after Alex joined ECI, Helen took a position with Telstar. Alex wanted analyses of the internal Telstar health care data set and Helen was the key. As a integral part of the Telstar negotiating team, she had been at his presentation to the executive board and had been impressed.

Table 5.3
Decreased Health Care Cost with Integrated Treatment of Substance Abuse–Related Medical Conditions

	Integrated* (N = 189)	Independent (N = 181)	
• **Annual cost decrease**	**$ 2,772**	**$708**	p < .02
Inpatient services	$1,920	$156	p < .04
Emergency room	$264	$252	p < .02
• **Abstinent 6 months**	**69%**	**55%**	p < .006

* Integrated primary care and chemical dependence services. *Note:* When substance-use disorder treatment is combined with general medical care in the medical setting for patients with physical complications of substance abuse, Parthasarathy and colleagues found that abstinence rates were higher and health care service use reduced compared to treatment in separate physical health and substance abuse programs.
Source: Adapted from S. Parthasarathy, J. Mertens, C. Moore, and C. Weisner, "Utilization and Cost Impact of Integrating Substance Abuse Treatment and Primary Care," *Medical Care* 41, no. 3 (2003): 357–67.

Part of Telstar's health contracts required that monthly aggregated employee physical health, mental health, and substance-use disorder service use be downloaded directly to an actuarial vendor-controlled, access-protected computer. The third-party vendor sheltered individual employee health information (personal health information, PHI) from Telstar management and its subsidiaries but allowed health use information to be linked to Family and Medical Leave Act (FMLA), short-term disability (STD), and long-term disability (LTD) data for Telstar's employees. A recent addition to the columns in the data set included use of case and disease management services, EAP, and health promotion.

Through this data warehouse, it was theoretically possible to compare the total cost of care, subcategorized into medical, pharmacy, and behavioral health service utilization, for employees categorized in several ways:

- Those entering STD and LTD versus those who did not.
- Those assisted by case and disease management versus sickness severity matched triggered employees who were not assisted.
- Those using EAP and/or health promotion services versus those who were offered the services but chose not to use them.

Helen was as compulsive as they come, and though she did not check and recheck that her front door had been locked, she did worry over details. Alex's request wrapped her up tight. "I can't be sure the data is clean. I could be sending you off with reports based on an inaccurate data dump."

Alex calmed her down, explaining that, at this point, he just wanted to confirm that the general information in the health reports he had recently studied meshed with Telstar's statistics. Specifically, did employees who used behavioral health services truly use twice as many medical services as those who did

not? Are the majority of antidepressant medications prescribed by nonpsychiatrists? Do behavioral health problems contribute substantially to STD and LTD
costs? Also helpful would be the impact of case and disease management on
worker performance and health care cost.

"Not an order too big for you, is it Helen?"

Her response was immediate. "Give me 10 of your staff and I'll have it to you
in no time."

* * *

Helen put two dedicated people to the task immediately. She knew what Alex
was up to and respected the direction he traveled. A recovering alcoholic, she
knew firsthand the troubles involved in accessing substance-use disorder treatment. For some, Alcoholics Anonymous worked, for others, like herself, it took
an intensive outpatient program. Though she had been sober for a long while,
she was still paying off the clinic bill. Even with Telstar's comprehensive health
coverage package, a relapse would rock her financial stability.

As the complex analyses rolled in confirming Alex's premise that medical and
pharmacy costs for employees tapping behavioral health service were high and related
to STD and LTD, Helen did a few of her own investigations. Nonpsychiatrists wrote
67 percent of all prescriptions for psychiatric medications (not only antidepressants).
In fact, 79 percent of discrete patients received their prescriptions from primary and
specialty physical health doctors, many of which were not refilled after the first.

Tracking two years of data downloads, she compared employees who used
chemical dependence and mental health services in year one with those who used
only medical services. In year two, the mental health and substance-use disorder
group that had three times the service use as those with only medical service use
in year one, but no use of chemical dependence or mental health services in year
two, showed reduced total service use near to that of those who used only physical health services. Those who continued to need both chemical dependence and
mental health services in year two increased total service use by about another
third compared to year one. Resolution of symptoms appeared to be associated
with significant cost reduction, persistence of symptoms with cost escalation.

Crunching the numbers, Helen figured very simplistically that Telstar could
conservatively save at least $1 million on health care costs for every 10 percent
of those insured by the company in which the ravages of psychiatric illness could
be reversed (psychiatrically ill = 20,250/135,000 [15%] employees plus family members × 0.1 × $500). An additional $1.35 million in lower absenteeism,
increased productivity, and reduced disability payments could be saved for every
10 percent of those with psychiatric illness in which mental health and substance-
use disorder problems were successfully addressed (9,000/60,000 [15%] × 0.1 ×
$1,500).[17] Because the vast majority of savings would be from decreases in physi-
cal health, not psychiatric, costs and enhanced productivity, such savings only
could be expected if behavioral health services were integrated with physical
health. More effective mental health and substance-use disorder treatment in the
current carved-out paradigm could not and would not have the same predictive
capabilities. Interaction of the worlds of physical and mental health was the key.

Further, it would contribute to reducing unnecessary administrative expenses of health care, which, in 1999, were calculated to account for nearly 31 percent of total health care spending, excluding health care industry personnel.[18]

Helen shared that she anticipated a minimum of 30 percent improvement in psychiatric and medical outcomes, an annual savings of $7.05 million in claims costs for Telstar employees ($564,000 for ECI alone). Her calculations were based on a crude macro look at medical service use and figures derived from published studies. She fully anticipated that as clinic-level integrated care changes were made, it would be possible to target complex, high-risk, high-cost employees, such as those with delirium, unexplained somatic complaints, both alcoholism and mental illness, autism, bipolar disorder, depression and anxiety associated with chronic medical conditions, and so forth, much more effectively. Integrated treatment of these patients, who are in the 10 percent who use 70 percent of resources (Figure 3.2), could be considered low-hanging fruit, reaping greater saving as they received improved care through integration.

Using an integrated prototype, which should be associated with far lower administrative costs for health plans once work processes had been established, breakeven would occur even sooner. Further, savings not only were accomplished but provided better care for employees rather than just saving money by limiting access and utilization. This was a win-win situation.

Based on his interviews and research, in combination with Helen's contribution, Alex arrived at the solid conclusion that mental health and substance-use disorder care needed to become a basic clinical and administrative component of general medical care: an integrated system in which all qualified practitioners would be supported through equitable reimbursement mechanisms in providing psychiatric services, regardless of clinical location. Perhaps more importantly, in the integrated setting that he envisioned, physical health clinicians would become as accountable for mental health and substance-use disorder outcomes as they were for physical problems. Behavioral health practitioners also would be responsible for helping improve outcomes for the physical disorders co-occurring with the emotional and behavioral problems they were addressing. Professionals from both disciplines would take ownership for total care of the patients they treated.

It was his hope that this would reverse the many situations in which human Ping-Pong was played. Whether the condition was physical or psychiatric, it no longer would be possible to refuse payment for services because of divisions in a health plan's network of physical and behavioral health providers. It would not matter if the services were provided in the physical or behavioral health setting. Patients suffering acute alcohol withdrawal symptoms while recovering from surgery for a bleeding ulcer in a medical setting would be able to initiate the process of alcoholism treatment during withdrawal and medical stabilization. Rehabilitation even may be offered in the medical setting. Treatment for medical complications of substance-use disorders would be just one part of the treatment of substance dependence, whether it is alcohol rehabilitation or methadone maintenance.

To accomplish health care integration would require disbanding the existing segregated physical health and mental health and substance-use disorder business structure that is inequitable and promotes the wrong kind of competition at the expense of good care. Medical benefits pay higher reimbursement rates with fewer authorization requirements and no accountability for improvement for general medical practitioners who choose to treat psychiatric illness despite a dismal success record without behavioral health assistance. Payment and benefit restrictions discourage, if not eliminate, mental health and substance-use disorder practitioner involvement in the medical setting even though psychiatric illness has a dramatic effect on both medical service use and outcomes.

Furthermore, independent medical and behavioral business practices delineate clinical responsibility and accountability along disciplinary lines. Even if payment and authorization practices were equivalent (parity), it would accomplish little because practitioners have learned well that responsibility for outcomes does not cross from medicine to psychiatry and vice versa. In the existing separation paradigm, passing the buck is encouraged and expected, which is a disservice to the patients treated, but mostly to those who remain ineffectively treated or untreated.

As Alex prepared his health service usage presentation for the meeting, he applied what he had learned about the symbiotic relationship of poor health care to high costs. He would advise a forward-thinking approach that would commit ECI-contracted health plans to gear their products toward integration. The contract would stipulate:

- Mandatory coordinated care by physical health physicians and their mental health and substance-use disorder colleagues in the physical health setting for all patients with complex and/or chronic illnesses.
- High-level communication between and among case and disease management support systems for physical and behavioral health at the health plan level with integrated clinical setting practitioners.
- Equitable reimbursement structures and strict adherence to parity regarding limit and restriction discrepancies between medical disciplines.
- Elimination of cost-shifting service utilization tactics.
- Quarterly and annual outcome reports documenting the value that health plans deliver to ECI through their integrated care and care management programs.

If the Blues, Medical Mart, Ecumenical Care, and their owned or subcontracted managed behavioral health organizations refused to retool to accommodate an integrated system in order to comply with ECI's (and Telstar's) stipulations, he would not hesitate to shop elsewhere. He had no doubts that the health plan that came up with the better mousetrap was in for a substantial increase in market share and a standing ovation from a citizenry weary of throwing good money into a bad system.

It was a bold plan—a gamble. But Polonius from the archives of English lit had taught Alex something valuable: "To thine own self be true." He knew he could not work for an industry he did not respect, an industry that divvied out benefits like a playground bully, "one for you, two for me," an industry that put profit before patients. While robbing the United States of good health care, someone was making a killing on the backs of worthy paying customers and quality health practitioners, and in that he wanted no part.

Colorado was in the light breezes of early summer when Alex presented his plan for health care integration, but he did not break a sweat.

Chapter 6

THE ALLIANCE FORMS

After you've done a thing the same way for two years, look it over carefully. After five years, look at it with suspicion. And after ten years, throw it away and start all over.[1]

—Alfred Edward Perlman

With an enthusiastic nod from Mr. Kishi and a guarded affirmation from the other board members, Alex put the pedal to the metal. He had until late fall to convince the Blues, Medical Mart, and Ecumenical Care that they were on the wrong page and to renegotiate their contracts. Within that time frame, if he failed to incite change, ECI would resume business as usual, with or without him. Alex knew that the challenges ahead were colossal and that he could not do it alone.

During the fact-finding odyssey in preparation for the ECI executive board meeting, Alex had interviewed a sampling of providers, four of whom he had befriended. Of like mind, each had pledged his or her support if Alex got the green light to pursue his objective of integration on all levels of health care.

Spencer was a hospital internist, and Tyler was a clinic-based family medicine physician. Austin and Heather were psychiatrists, general adult and child, respectively. Though from competing but collaborative clinic systems, all four participated in administrative decision-making and were considered thought leaders in their fields. Alex also wanted input from Jeff, the chief operations officer for University Hospitals and Clinics. He was directly involved in the administration of health services for the local university hospital and had previously worked for the Providence Hospital System, a regional powerhouse.

To be fully prepared to field arguments from the health plan administrators, Alex called on these five to provide a blueprint on regional general medical

and behavioral health care availability and the components that went into decisions about what clinical services were and were not offered to ECI and Telstar
employees. Spencer took the lead in arranging a casual Sunday brunch meeting
at his condo, where interruptions would be few. While Spencer folded chilies into
omelets, Alex pitched questions.

GENERAL MEDICAL AND BEHAVIORAL HEALTH
CLINICAL SERVICES

Compared to other metropolitan areas, there was nothing special about health
care delivery in Denver. Mental health and substance-use disorder services were
provided in independent clinics and on administratively autonomous inpatient
units. Little or no communication existed between the physical and behavioral
health practitioners even though they were taking care of the same patients. Physical health and mental health/substance-use disorder clinical notes, consultation
reports, and testing results for patients were stored either in separate data warehouses or on the same electronic server restricted by a firewall from clinicians
outside of their discipline, even though the clinicians may be taking care of health
problems in the same patient. Several hospitals and clinics used ECI's Version
6.02 electronic medical record, the latest to undergo beta testing. Discounted for
local delivery systems, it had many bells and whistles.

Jeff noted that for the past year and a half Ecumenical Care had sponsored a
psychiatric nurse case manager in one university medical clinic that treated a high
percentage of its very ill, largely indigent and elderly enrollees. Without the Ecumenical Care grant, the case manager would have needed to be subsidized from
the clinic's per diem and income by the general practitioners because Ferdinand
Behavioral (FB) reimbursement for services was small and complicated to collect
since the service was provided in a medical setting. To charge FB for case management services, all patient encounters required preauthorization. Jeff had not
heard about outcomes in terms of patient care improvements or cost reduction but
understood that Ecumenical Care was presently measuring the effect of what they
called *integrated services.*

Heather and Austin confirmed that Colorado had a shortage of psychiatrists and
other behavioral health specialists in 43 of its 64 counties. Denver was not listed
among them. Few psychiatrists in Denver, however, were inclined to provide consultation services in the inpatient setting or engage in outpatient collaborative
care in the physical health settings because authorization procedures were more
onerous and reimbursement more limited than in the psychiatric setting. Further,
health plan regulations prevented two different providers from billing for patient
visits on the same day. These rules defeated the purpose of having a psychiatrist
on-site to support the primary care physicians and their patients because their
services would not be reimbursed.

It also was clear that the payers intended for psychiatrists to limit their services
to 15-minute so-called medication checks in psychiatric clinics despite the cost
efficacy in combining psychotherapy and medication management.[2] Payment

rates for those services allowed the highest return for time spent, thus office administrators maximized clinic profits by filling their psychiatrists' days with 15-minute appointments. Such short visits, however, did not do much for the psychiatrists' relationships with their patients. It also earned them the bristling reputation for being pill pushers by both their physical health and mental health and substance-use disorder colleagues.

Heather and Austin were not aware of any changes in reimbursement mechanisms or amounts for services given in the physical health setting from any of ECI's health plans in the past three years. In fact, there had been a slow but steady exodus of what both Austin and Heather considered excellent psychiatrists, and especially child psychiatrists, from the behavioral health networks that serviced ECI, whether insourced (carved-in) as psychiatric care was with the Blues or carved out to BVD and FB as Ecumenical Care and Medical Mart did.

Recognizing that managed behavioral health organization (MBHO) business practices were prejudicial and detrimental to their patients, many psychiatrists were choosing to opt out of behavioral health networks. Rather, they would see direct-pay patients and avoid the red tape and the 15-minute medication check demands. Because up to two-thirds of mental health and substance-use disorder contracts had a 50 percent, rather than a 20 percent, co-pay requirement that was still allowed in Employee Retirement Income Security Act (ERISA) self-insured health plan contracts even in parity states, the cost difference of in-network and out-of-network services was insignificant to most patients. Psychiatrists also were dropping out of Medicare and Medicaid provider networks, leaving a skeletal staff to treat the sickest and most needy patients, most of whom were elderly, uninsured, or assigned to public programs because of complex high-cost illness.

Though Heather and Austin were not among them, they did know several colleagues who had a special interest in caring for physically ill patients with psychiatric disorders. Willing to take the financial hit, these psychiatrists had tried to organize mental health and substance-use disorder teams in the physical health setting. General medical administrators, however, who stated perfunctorily that their clinics would lose money if they agreed to add the services, stopped these endeavors cold. If and when they had available space, they preferentially supported other medical specialty practitioners, particularly those who offered procedures that generated the most income, such as cardiologists, gastroenterologists, orthopedists, and so forth.

The story was the same for psychiatrists and their internist colleagues interested in providing high-acuity integrated inpatient services in the physical health setting. Despite a well-recognized need for general medical beds with psychiatric capabilities, general hospitals, even those with imbedded general hospital psychiatric units, shied away from coordinating physical and mental health/substance-use disorder care in the same setting. Discharge and readmission requirements for patients with concurrent illness were hassle enough.

Furthermore, reimbursement for psychiatric admissions was far less than for general hospital or medical specialty admissions, and patient stays were longer. On the few occasions patients with concurrent illness were admitted, the financial outcome was disastrous. Locked in a standoff as to who was responsible for the bill, not infrequently neither behavioral nor general medical health plans paid for the services. The hospital was left with an unpaid bill and a patient at risk of bankruptcy as hospitals tried to collect.

Spencer and Tyler agreed that getting psychiatric consultations for their patients in the medical setting was nearly impossible. Their only alternative was to refer the 10 percent to 20 percent of their patients who needed mental health and substance-use disorder assistance, but the typical wait for an adult psychiatry appointment was 4 to 12 weeks and for child psychiatry 12 to 24 weeks.[3] With delays like these, fewer than half of Spencer's and Tyler's patients showed up for their scheduled appointments. Of those who did, only half returned for recommended follow-up visits. Without supervision, few adhered to treatment. Spencer estimated maybe 1 in 20 of his patients benefited from a psychiatric referral, not from lack of efficacy of psychiatric treatment, but because of the system hassles of getting the patient to an appropriate specialist in a timely fashion.

Even though fund administrators tout a shift toward integrating behavioral and general health care in their plans, all agreed that they knew of no health plans particularly interested in addressing the needs of patients with combined physical and mental health problems, nor of any change in authorization or reimbursement procedures that led to improved patient care. Jeff confirmed that as a decision-maker regarding the type of programs that his university system might consider in the next several years, integrated physical and mental health clinics and inpatient units had not been discussed. He said that there had not been active consideration about improving the shortage of psychiatrists (adult, child, geriatric, or emergency room), psychologists, psychiatric nurse clinicians, or psychiatric beds. Reimbursement was inadequate to support development of any of these services despite tremendous clinical need.

* * *

At home later that evening, Alex consolidated the information gleaned from the Sunday meeting and contemplated his game plan. He had learned that fund distributors were complicated organisms, and as king of the mountain they were going to dig in their heels to maintain the status quo within their own industry.

Though available in an array of shapes and sizes, all health plans have similar basic components. They have a board of directors and an executive staff, composed of a chief executive officer (CEO), chief operating officer (COO), chief financial officer (CFO), and chief medical officer (CMO), surrounded by a bevy of vice presidents. The vice presidents divvy up the real work performed in health plan departments, including marketing and sales, network management, contract writing, customer and provider services, care management (utilization management, case management, disease management, appeals, etc.), information technology, and claims processing. Contract benefit descriptions are based on actuarial projections derived from prior physical health business with clients subclassified in numerous ways, such as commercial; public programs (Medicaid); seniors (Medicare); large, medium, and small businesses; fully insured (health plans at risk for claims expenses with state and federal regulated coverage mandates) and self-insured (large employers at risk for claims expenses, but fewer coverage mandates); among others.

To put forward their best foot they have a public relations staff backed up by a number of lawyers. Quality assurance staff perform assessments of their network providers' credentials and performance in selected clinical domains. Finally, the organization is held together as any other business by a human resources staff who cater to the needs of the organization and its employees.

Mental health and substance-use disorder coverage, considered distinct from general medical health coverage, has its own duplicated organizational infrastructure virtually identical to that of the physical health component of the business. For some, like Ecumenical Care and Medical Mart, the behavioral health infrastructure is independently owned (BVD and FB) and completely disconnected from the physical health business, though the two support services for the same patients and communicate to the degree necessary to keep them and their members out of trouble. For others, like the Blues, behavioral health business is a separate subsection of the company. Like with the carve-outs, it has an independent administrative structure and work processes, including customer service, care management, and claims adjudication. Mental health and substance-use disorder service use is analyzed separately from physical health for purposes of actuarial projections. Importantly, payment for behavioral health assessment and treatment comes from a completely segregated bottom line: same structure, different management.

Alert to the resource hemorrhage resulting from ineffective and misdirected health care service use, fund distributors have recently attempted to rescript policies to address conspicuous inadequacies in supporting care for members with both physical and mental health difficulties. Stirring vigorous discussion recently is that mental illness now constitutes a major contributor to disease burden in the United States both in human and economic terms.[4] With approximately 30 percent of adult Americans suffering from at least one mental disorder and less than one-third of them receiving any kind of help, the pressure is on.

To date, all responses have been made without tinkering with either the physical health or the mental health and substance-use disorder business management practices. Fund distributors suggest that they are coordinating general medical and behavioral health services by paying primary care physicians to treat depression. They also set up hotlines to mental health and substance-use disorder clinicians or on-site counselors for selected primary care clinics to improve mental health support access.

Unfortunately, the information Alex collected during the discussion at Spencer's, if accurate, indicates that actual behavioral health access falls far short of the promises of integrated health care made by the health plans. Hotlines may be available, but who is going to call into a black box for help? On-site counselors are available only in boutique medical practices and are certainly not widespread. Tyler said his clinic looked into adding the service but decided it was economically impossible without subsidy. Jeff confirmed that the psychiatric nurse case manager in their university medical clinic would cost them extra without the Ecumenical Care subsidy.

He commented, however, that early reports suggest that patients do better when case management is available.

ASKING HARD QUESTIONS ABOUT INTEGRATED PHYSICAL HEALTH AND MENTAL HEALTH/ SUBSTANCE-USE DISORDER CARE

Monday morning, Alex requested independent appointments with key representatives at the Blues, Medical Mart, and Ecumenical Care, with the intent of clarifying how each of them integrated physical health and psychiatric services. Specifically, he was looking for direct and honest answers to five questions:

1. How do health plan benefits facilitate primary and specialty medical care physicians' ability to collaborate and coordinate treatment for ECI and Telstar employees and their dependents with mental health and substance-use disorder specialists for psychiatric needs in the medical setting and vice versa?

2. How does total cost of care subcategorized into physical health, pharmacy, and behavioral health service utilization for ECI and Telstar employees and family members who used mental health and substance-use disorder services compare to those who used only physical health services?

3. How do ECI's health plan benefits encourage mental health and substance-use disorder professionals to practice in primary and specialty physical health care clinic settings? The inpatient corollary to this is how do they support the development, use, and maintenance of units capable of actively addressing concurrent physical and psychiatric illness in the same location for complex patients?

4. What percentage of ECI and Telstar employees and dependents are assisted by the coordinated and internally consistent efforts of physical health and psychiatric case and disease managers? What percentage of enrollees use each/both, and how does care management help change outcomes in comparison to matched patients who are not offered or refuse it?

5. In what percentage of employees and dependents entering disease management for diabetes, asthma, and heart disease does a depression-screening tool identify depression? How are those with a concurrent depression assisted?

He briefly explained in a blanket e-mail to account representatives at the Blues, Ecumenical Care, and Medical Mart that ECI and Telstar were actively pursuing a review of the effectiveness of health care delivery to their employees. Results of the review would be used during health plan renegotiations in the fall.

Other than planting a bee in their bonnets, Alex did not expect to accomplish much in these initial contacts. He was not disappointed. Within three days, he met with the Blues' account rep, and before her briefcase was out of hand, Julie quickly assured Alex that they currently insourced behavioral health care and that ECI was receiving the best and most forward-thinking integrated product on the market.

Because the Blues owned their own behavioral health product, he had presumed they would be in an advantageous position to meet his demands but learned in an on-site review of the Blues' work flows with Spencer and Jeff that whether owned or not, the Blues' behavioral health was, for all practical purposes, as carved-out as the other two health plans ECI used. Customer and provider services and care management functions were performed by independent groups of physical health and mental health professionals located on separate floors and to some extent in separate buildings. Utilization management staff used two noncommunicating sets of medical-necessity criteria and independent software documentation systems. General medical and behavioral services had disparate prior and retrospective authorization procedures and case management capabilities.

Though they issued one card, members called different numbers from the backs of their insurance cards to get assistance. In fact, the Blues had some accounts that purchased only their physical but not behavioral health products, and vice versa. There were no other core physical health disciplines, such as cardiology, ophthalmology, radiology, and so forth within their suite of offerings in which customers could opt out when purchasing care. In short, the Blues' psychiatric business had its own bottom line. It had its own benefit definitions and distinctive contract clauses, its own network of providers and credentialing process. It had its own claims-processing algorithms and data warehouse. Communication occurred only in crisis cases.

As Alex presented facts about what he meant by integration of physical and behavioral health to Julie, she had not flinched. When he finished, she reiterated that she was dead sure most purchasers of the Blues' plans, including ECI and Telstar, negotiated rates through one health care contract and paid one monthly premium for the physical and behavioral care combination, which translated into the best coordination of services possible.

Without comment, Alex handed Julie a hard copy of the presentation he had given at the recent ECI executive board meeting and the list of five questions he had sent her earlier in e-mail correspondence when requesting a meeting. Emphasizing findings from the Goetzel report (Table 5.2),[5] which showed that psychiatric disorders contributed substantially to ECI's and Telstar's total health related costs, he asked her to find out what the Blues were going to do to meet his objectives. "Give me a heads up when you've got the answers."

At his meeting with Medical Mart and their behavioral health contractor, FB, Alex was somewhat pushed off balance with their complete lack of interest in considering a new approach to integrating behavioral health. Melanie, the Medical Mart representative, clarified early in the discussion that the focal point of their enterprise was supporting physical health services. Though she did not specifically say it, she implied that mental health and substance-use disorder services, though necessary, were inconvenient expenses best handled by management business practices that limit access and service. In less than a half-hour, the meeting disbanded. Alex left the same package on the table and the same injunction, "Give me a call when you've had time to look over the material." To retain a lucrative account, no doubt, he would hear back from them, but begrudgingly.

Curiously, at Ecumenical Care, Alex was directed to the office of the vice president of operations, a step up from the customary account liaison. Extending his hand to Alex, Edward introduced himself and said, "You are the wave maker, I presume?"

The answer came quiet and firm. "I believe so."

Edward explained that for reasons not yet public, BVD, their behavioral health arm, would not attend the meeting as Alex had requested. He informed Alex that he and the CEO of Ecumenical Care, Mr. Romani, had reviewed with great interest ECI's questionnaire and were eager to learn more. "With exorbitant health care premiums now driving employers out of business, we've seen the train coming," he said.

Over the next couple of hours, Alex learned that Ecumenical Care already had taken initial steps to transition to an integrated system. They now downloaded mental health and substance-use disorder claims data from BVD to their own system servers and were in the process of consolidating the data with their own physical health claims. Having read about the same integrated outpatient models that Alex had, Ecumenical Care already had inserted a psychiatric nurse test case manager in a primary care clinic at the university hospital on an experimental basis. Because Ecumenical Care had a high percentage of members in this clinic, the case manager was liberally working with medical case managers at the health plan and disease managers at AdvancedDM to achieve better total health improvement for clinic patients.

Ecumenical Care anticipated that this partnership would lead to lower medical service use for their enrollees. When both a chronic illness and depression were present, the clinic case manager made sure AdvancedDM disease managers were involved. In coordination with the clinic primary care physicians, she also frequently encouraged referral of patients to cognitive behavioral therapists, a psychiatrist, and/or consulted with the Ecumenical Care psychiatrist medical director to ensure that the right medications were being given when patients did not seem to be improving and referral was not possible.

Though stressing the transition to authentic integrated care and eliminating BVD had not yet been announced, Edward all but assured Alex that Ecumenical Care was on board. Unlike the Blues and Medical Mart, Edward and Mr. Romani had done their homework and understood the efforts restructuring would entail. Alex breathed a sigh of relief that at least one of ECI's health plans was ready to push the boundaries. As Alex prepared to leave, Edward fished a business card out of his wallet and urged Alex to give Dr. Vicki a call. "Bets are on she'll be an asset in your crusade to bring about change."

THE CARVE-IN (BLUES)

Gathered around trays of melon wedges and muffins, the top dogs of the Blues' management teams grumbled at the interruption. Most in attendance agreed Alex's outlandish mission did not have a prayer. A few were not so sure. Though ECI was a small potato in their commercial business, if Alex had a hook into the parent company Telstar, as it appeared he did, the loss would be treacherous. He was no lightweight. As president-elect of the Mid-Colorado Coalition of Businesses, his influence could not be underestimated.

Although the Blues now owned their mental health and substance-use disorder business, management practices for behavioral health were virtually identical to carved-out managed care companies. Benefit language was adapted from a number of managed behavioral health contracts from previous years. The task force assigned to address Alex's requests began the meeting to discuss in detail each of the five questions. How did the Blues score?

Questions 1 and 3: Benefit descriptions encourage physical health and mental health/substance-use disorder practitioner and care coordination in a single setting (grade C–):

- Benefits did not change when the Blues insourced behavioral health care. Payment was still from a separate pool of money, and that bottom line was scrutinized closely. Member and provider contracts did nothing new to encourage or support psychiatric services in the physical health setting or physical health services in the mental health and substance-use disorder settings, whether inpatient or outpatient.

- The transition to an insourced behavioral health product did allow greater internal control (and slightly lower administrative cost) because the Blues: (1) now ran its own mental health and substance-use disorder provider network and credentialing process; (2) information systems had an independent but parallel mental health and substance-use disorder claims adjudication process; (3) customer and provider queries were handled by service staff with similar training and work processes, though from independent locations and with different staff-to-member ratios (lower for behavioral health); (4) utilization and case management was handled separately but internally; and (5) actuarial staff were able to directly determine independent mental health and substance-use disorder contract risk profiles.

Question 2: Subcategorized total health cost reporting, which assesses care management value (grade D):

- It is not possible to compare members with behavioral health service use to those using only medical services because behavioral health claims were stored in a completely separate server. To consolidate data sets would take anywhere from three to six months if the project was put at the top of an already extensive work request priority list.

Question 4: Outcomes with case and disease management (grade D):

- Consolidated reports for members using physical and behavioral health case and disease management services would have to be done by hand because the care manager documentation system for each does not capture care management entries. There was also no ongoing record to track members accepting or rejecting case management assistance.

- Case management procedures by mental health and substance-use disorder staff differed from physical health staff. Mental health and substance-use disorder staff worked directly with the providers of high-cost behavioral health patients to adjudicate when care was appropriate. Physical health case managers worked primarily with the patients and their families to facilitate best practices and physical health care coordination.

- Nurses specializing in complex physically ill patients talked with nurses assigned to high-cost psychiatric patients more frequently than in the past. The process, however, remained hit-and-miss because the care management medical and psychiatric health documentation systems did not communicate.

Question 5: Integrated disease management (grade D):

- Patients with chronic illnesses entering or refusing disease management were recorded in the AdvancedDM database, but the Blues would have to formally request a customized report that compared outcomes. AdvancedDM did not screen their clients for depression.

The room fell silent. It was crystal clear to all that the Blues had not and could not deliver functional health care integration to ECI using its current paradigm. To do so would require a disruptive and costly dismantling of not only their Blues Behavioral product but also the entire current health care infrastructure. Although insourcing behavioral health associated with internal cost savings due to administrative consolidation, it was evident that there was no documentable real value brought to ECI. No time to waste, they rolled up their sleeves and went to work on projections for strategic realignment that they would present at the follow-up meeting with Alex.

THE CARVE-OUT (MEDICAL MART/FB)

The partnership of medical care organizations (MCOs) with MBHOs, like Ecumenical Care/BVD and Medical Mart/FB, were surprisingly similar to the insoured Blues model in their ability to integrate care. All were far from praiseworthy. Because Ecumenical Care had felt the tremors of change for some time and had poised for it, they had little reviewing to do to answer Alex's questionnaire. Medical Mart and FB had just begun. Sans a formal task force presentation, the account representatives, Melanie from Medical Mart and Michael from FB, held a roundtable discussion to prepare for the follow-up meeting with Alex.

FB's provider network had substantially decreased in size due to rigid authorization procedures, work site demands, and disparities in reimbursement rates to the actual cost of practice experienced by psychiatrists, child psychiatrists, and doctoral psychologists. As long as Michael did not update FB's list of network providers, they appeared to be in compliance with state and federal access requirements to have an adequate number of providers in each geographic area to serve enrollees. In fact, they were below standards even in nonshortage areas.

There was little chance, however, that discrepancies in provider access would be uncovered because patients (members) called for appointments individually. Difficulties would occur in identifying a clinician to help their enrollees, but there was little likelihood that patients would talk with each other and publicize the shortage. Everyone knew there were too few providers anyhow. Michael also made sure that patients always could get an appointment with a master's level counselor, which counted as fulfilling the requirement for access. Michael reasoned that if a patient really needed to see a psychiatrist, there was always the emergency room—a safety net up and running 24 hours a day.

The limited psychiatrist and doctorate-level psychologist network actually worked to FB's economic advantage because it meant a lower number of their enrollees would use high-cost providers. Because FB did not typically pay for the bulk of emergency room visits, it was a big win. Premiums for the behavioral health component of health care could be held in check.

Unfortunately, a shortage of qualified network providers also meant that those most likely to effect outcome change in a patient's condition were not available to care for them. Counselors are helpful for personal and social crisis intervention and support. They, however, can not provide outcome-changing treatment for psychosis, major depression, mania, anxiety disorder, attention-deficit/hyperactivity disorder (ADHD), eating disorders, autism, somatization, delirium, substance abuse, dementia, and many other psychiatric illnesses without the involvement of a specialist with a higher level of mental health or substance-use disorder expertise. But this was not FB's problem.

As with the Blues, health care service use documentation (claims processing) for physical (Medical Mart) and mental health/substance-use disorders (FB) were performed in independent computer systems. FB owned the behavioral health data. It had no agreement to share it with Medical Mart. Even if FB was willing to share this information with Medical Mart, patient identifiers in the two data sets did not correspond. Therefore, Melanie could and would give cost analyses for physical health service use and Michael for mental health and substance-use disorder service use, but there would be no combined analyses. Alex would just have to get over it.

Case management for psychiatric conditions was provided in the FB call center, located in California, though Medical Mart was in Colorado. Managers at the two sites talked rarely because privacy issues were paramount to Melanie and Michael. Most of the time, Medical Mart and FB case managers did not realize that another case manager also was assisting the client with whom they were working.

Medical Mart and FB managers performed their management functions very differently. Medical Mart mainly used certified nurse case managers to work directly with the top 0.5 percent of the enrollees who triggered a new predictive modeling algorithm. This was well below the 1 percent to 2 percent national benchmark, but few purchasers knew to ask. True to case management principles, medical case managers helped patients identify the best care in an increasingly complex system and halved health care service use in pre/post analyses.

FB case managers, on the other hand, were selected from a pool of utilization managers with social work and licensed counseling backgrounds. Few had nursing degrees or experience. They performed what they called case management on a small but unknown percentage of patients with high behavioral health service utilization. Before they started, these case managers received a half-day seminar on what FB considered case management before they went to work. Consistent with their training, they exclusively worked through the patients' clinicians. They did not talk with patients. There was no attempt by FB to establish value, and neither Medical Mart nor FB compared outcomes for those who received their brands of case management with common patients who triggered positive in each system.

Like the Blues, FB was not able to give information about depression disease management screening in patients with chronic physical illnesses. AdvancedDM and FB disease management activities were separate. Staff in each did not talk with one another. They did not even know which employees worked with managers from both. Michael was pleased, however, that the issue had surfaced because it meant that next year he may be able to sell an expanded stand-alone yet coordinated depression disease management product for all of Telstar employees. Michael did not realize how far off base he was.

Despite aggressively and independently managing physical and mental health/ substance-use disorder care, Medical Mart and FB both recognized that integration was increasingly being demanded by their accounts. As a means of biding time while they made necessary adjustments, they redoubled their message. "Only through utilization management of mental health and substance-use disorder benefits by MBHOs could purchasers of health care packages expect to control the behavioral health care dollar." They downplayed the data that showed that what they encouraged merely shifted costs to physical health benefits (Figure 5.5).

Interim solutions to the drumbeat for integration took the form of educating primary care physicians in the treatment of depression and encouraging screens for depression in the primary care setting. To further assist primary care physicians deal with depression, they provided 24-hour 800-number access to a psychiatrist or psychologist. The call-in number was not a referral line. It was a help line for primary care physicians willing to treat behavioral health patients themselves. FB also added contract mandates that its behavioral health network members accept next-day referrals for Medical Mart enrollees, regardless of whether there was a full clinic schedule. Though this tactic did not endear them to the few psychiatrist and psychologist network participants who remained, this was their solution to quell the patient demands for timely access.

With their current application of behavioral health care shining a less than favorable light on Medical Mart/FB's ability to provide Alex the kind of health care integration he expected, Melanie and Michael began the tedious task of figuring out how they might comply. Unbeknownst to them, Alex's grades for the Medical Mart/FB combo to his questions were all Fs.

                                    * * *

As the health plans feverishly worked toward accommodating Alex, Alex followed up on Edward's lead and called Dr. Vicki. With a national and international reputation as a leader in integrated care and well connected with physicians who were at the leading edge of research, she would prove an invaluable asset to Alex's efforts.

An internist and psychiatrist with 20 years' experience in integrated clinical care, Vicki had recently moved to Denver with her husband and three children to accept a position in the Providence hospital system. She had been specifically recruited to implement steps to improve the hospital's delivery of psychiatric services. Providence, which managed more than 2,000 beds in several hospitals and numerous multispecialty clinics in the Denver region, had just been sued for negligence after one of its depressed general hospital medical patients had killed himself by stuffing toilet paper down his throat.

Jason had been hospitalized for alcohol-related pancreatitis on the medical unit. A psychiatrist consultation had been ordered two days prior to the suicide, but no one was available until week's end. Jason's doctors were aware that he was depressed and had assigned him a round-the-clock nurse to make sure he did not attempt anything. Because his condition required intravenous feeding and close medical monitoring, Jason could not be discharged from the general hospital and admitted to the psychiatric unit, though they were in the same building. Even if he could have been transferred, the family had made it clear that psychiatric care had to be discreet.

Out of nursing school only three years and with no experience in assisting with suicidal patients, the specials nurse had stepped out to get a bite to eat at the cafeteria after checking out with the unit charge nurse. She told the charge nurse that Jason had gone into the bathroom. Fifteen minutes later, the charge nurse found Jason dead, mouth and throat filled with toilet paper.

The charge nurse and specials nurse were devastated. Their inexperience was named in the legal action. Two years before Jason's death, a similar incident had occurred at another of the Providence hospitals, which further strengthened the legal case against them. As a condition to accepting the job at Providence, Vicki had demanded that a medical psychiatry unit[6] be established in Providence General, the anchor hospital for the system. Twice burned, Mr. Cooper, the CEO of the Providence system, was desperate, and because Vicki appeared to know what she was doing, the board agreed to her requirement.

HEALTH PLAN REPORTS

Official meetings with the ECI health plans took place with Julie representing the Blues; Melanie and Michael, Medical Mart and FB; and Edward, Ecumenical Care. They each reported their responses to Alex's questionnaire. With the exception of Ecumenical Care, the health plans had taken no serious steps to upgrade the coordination of general medical and behavioral health services.

At each meeting, the principals at the health plans concurred that the current health care system was not designed to integrate general medical and behavioral health care. The Blues in concert with Medical Mart and FB emphasized that it would be very expensive to change, requiring rewritten provider and member contracts, altering network credentialing and participants, merging claims processing, consolidating care management, just to name a few. It also would negate savings opportunities generated from the control measures designed to ensure that no behavioral health funds were used to support unnecessary and/or excessive behavioral health services. This, they argued, only could occur when behavioral health was segregated from the rest of medical care. Neither mentioned that the denial rates based on utilization review were at the 0.5 percent to 1 percent level.

It was far more expensive to hire staff to do the reviews than were the savings from denials.

Alex's concern was about the total cost of care rather than the behavioral health budget. He wanted to know how they proposed to increase the percentage of ECI and Telstar employees who received effective treatment for depression, substance-use disorders, and other psychiatric conditions that were associated with employee suffering, high general medical service use, employee absenteeism, disability, and low productivity. Emphasizing that study after study suggested the current system merely shifted costs from the behavioral to the medical budgets, he was interested in hearing their take on the situation from that angle.

Julie noted that the Blues were taking steps to increase the interaction of their physical health and mental health/substance-use disorder case managers, which should improve outcomes for some of the most complex and expensive patients by helping them get both the medical and psychiatric help they needed. Notably, Julie said nothing about contract redesign, network changes, and so forth. Further, there was no indication about how the case managers would promote coordination of care in a divided clinical system.

Melanie and Michael reinforced that Medical Mart and FB would be expanding education for primary care physicians about the treatment of depression and anxiety. Phone access to mental health and substance-use disorder specialists for primary and specialty physical health clinicians would be better publicized because few used the service at present. They intended to explore inserting more behavioral health specialists into selected multispecialty clinics as a quality improvement project and were researching ways to support access to psychiatric services in general hospital emergency rooms and on the inpatient units. Perhaps they could decrease the prior-authorization requirement for psychiatric consultants from before the first visit to after the second, making it less onerous for the consultant. They also recognized a need to reexamine a consultant's fee basis.

"This was a thorny issue," they told Alex, because it would involve expanding behavioral health related expenses and likely drive up premiums. Michael assured Alex that FB would do everything in its power to hold down the costs of this transition. He also noted that as the system process changes were being considered, ECI might wish to consider their new depression disease management product for all of ECI and Telstar's employees because it was being rolled out at a very competitive price.

Alex did not arrange a formal meeting with Edward. Instead they had a meeting of the minds over lunch during which Edward restated that very shortly Ecumenical Care would cut ties with BVD and handle its own behavioral health management. Although he was not at liberty to provide all the details about what was entailed, Edward noted that they had every intention of expanding and coordinating physical and psychiatric care internally. Externally, they also were considering ways to encourage the integration of physical health and mental health/substance-use disorder care at the clinical level. Independently, under Edward's leadership, the Strategic Planning Committee at Ecumenical Care had come to the same conclusion that had inspired Alex to call for change.

In business for nearly ten years, Ecumenical Care served a mixed account pool of nearly 300,000 members, and to introduce the changes within a manageable administrative infrastructure was feasible. They also had enough experience to do it in a systematic and thoughtful way. Moving forward, psychiatric treatment would be a core component of general medical health at Ecumenical Care.

Edward shared that insourcing of behavioral health was the first step.[7] As they did so, some programs would be introduced right away, such as expanding the medical provider network to include mental health and substance-use disorder personnel and building the customer service and care management support services as a part of existing general medical work processes. Selling psychiatric services as an integral part of all of their health care contracts would be a key component. There would be no mental health and substance-use disorder health exclusions, just as there were no cardiology and oncology exclusions.

The second stage would be to create a benefit set in which mental health and substance-use disorder services would be included as a part of other medical benefits. This would allow them to consolidate claims processing for physical and behavioral health services. The mental health and substance-use disorders funding pool would be folded into the medical, thereby eliminating the division. With this rearrangement, behavioral health benefit adjudication would require no special processing. From a practical standpoint, it would allow mental health and substance-use disorder specialists to practice and be paid regardless of clinical setting. It also would abandon the need to discharge and readmit inpatients when they transferred from general medicine or surgical units to psychiatry units. In fact, it would open the door to the development of inpatient treatment units that could address the needs of complex patients with concurrent and interacting physical and psychiatric illness.

From Edward's perspective, stages one and two required commitment by a base of purchasers who would see the process through as they partnered with Ecumenical Care to develop an approach to general medical and behavioral health integration. This, however, was to be a hurdle. Though fairly far along in the planning, they did not yet have a purchaser partner that would insure business solvency as they instituted rather remarkable, if not revolutionary, changes in the way they handled support for physical and psychiatric care.

Edward felt confident a partner would step up but noted that even with the best intentions of ECI, Telstar, and other purchasers in collaboration with Ecumenical Care, the project was doomed to failure if it was not coupled with change at the clinical level. It was on the examining table or at the hospital bedside that the rubber hit the road. Improved clinical, functional, and financial outcomes would not occur unless patients were treated better.

This was perhaps the greatest challenge. Edward wanted to involve clinical settings that were used most often by Ecumenical Care members, and these clinical settings would have to want to work with the health plan to effect change on behalf of the patients. Typically sitting on opposite sides of the bargaining table, the relationship between clinical operations and health plans was contentious and, therefore, collaboration between them and the providers that delivered their services a big if.

Finally, Edward noted that Ecumenical Care's plan likely would be the only health plan in the region to offer integrated services, at least initially. This obviously created problems for the clinical settings as they decided whether to collaborate in the initiative. For instance, University Hospitals did not restrict their services to Ecumenical Care enrollees. If they created integrated physical health and mental health/substance-use disorder clinics in the medical setting and/or medical psychiatry units in their hospitals, they would need some assurance that reimbursement by other fund distributors would be adequate to cover their costs and generate profit. Without this, the whole initiative was a nonstarter.

Alex was impressed. Edward obviously had given a lot of thought to how this would work. On the operational side, he was much farther along than Alex was. In fact, Edward's practical understanding of the health plan industry and description of the transition process underscored for Alex the complexity of his request to the other health plans. Never once did Alex question whether it was the right thing to do, but he did appreciate the enormity of the task.

NEXT STEPS

Alex did not kid himself that his proposal would materialize overnight. He had learned enough from Edward to know that the transition would have to be one bleacher at a time. Medical managed care organizations would have to let their multiyear subcontracts with the carved-out behavioral health vendors run out. Putting together the internal processes to make the transition, either with the help of companies springing up to help MCOs create their own internal behavioral health capabilities or with newly hired staff, would take time to complete the process toward health care integration. To sustain the forward momentum, he also would have to interest one or two major employers in the region to sign on with ECI and Telstar in order to put pressure on other medical health plans to emulate Ecumenical Care's advances. Luckily, after a charged presentation by Mr. Kishi to the Telstar board of directors, they were in.

It was now late November. ECI with Telstar would drop Medical Mart as a health plan. The Blues would be retained with the clear mandate that they were on notice to reconfigure integration of their services. Employees would be indirectly encouraged to consider Ecumenical Care as their health plan through signing incentives for the coming year. Already, several major employers in the Mid-Colorado Business Coalition were discussing health care contracts similar to Telstar's with their health plans. All fund distributors, including Ecumenical Care, would be expected to show the value of their management programs to enrollees through a reorganized reporting system.

Within the five months given to him by the executive board at ECI, Alex had loosed the boat from its moorings, and sails were up. Contracting would change but, more importantly, health care services to employees would improve. Edward's understanding of and solid commitment to seeing the introduction of integrated care become a reality was a major asset. Vicki's involvement in implementation at the clinical level, however, would define their success. With Alex at the helm, ECI was on its way.

Chapter 7

CLINICAL INTEGRATION

> If you have built castles in the air, your work need not be lost; that is
> where they should be. Now put foundations under them.[1]
>
> —Henry David Thoreau

Alex and Edward knew from the get-go that no matter how hard their efforts, success was not guaranteed. Without a firm commitment from Ecumenical Care, the goal to integrate health care was dead in the water, and though the company was determined to participate, it was a small health plan with limited influence in the region. Edward noted that participants providing integrated services would need to be paid by all the fund distributors in such a way as to make it profitable for them. If Ecumenical Care was the only health plan that supported mental health and substance-use disorder services in the medical setting, then few providers would develop programs. Start-up costs were significant and financial risks high.

Edward also worried that if Ecumenical Care was, in fact, to be the only health plan that created innovative integrated services, their upgraded services would attract foremost a large percentage of high-use/low-paying customers. Although there was the potential to capture a larger market share in three to five years, they also could be out of business because of adverse selection of enrollees. Edward was not sure that he could persuade the executives at Ecumenical Care to take the plunge.

Another barrier was the exhaustive measures needed to implement integrated care at the clinical level where it actually did its work. Alex and Edward had read many articles on how it could be done but had never seen it in operation. Familiar with the early studies showing that adding psychiatric services in the general medical setting did not lead to cost offset, they were all too aware that no hospital would willingly pay more to reap minimal or limited benefits for general medical and psychiatric integration. Luckily, Edward had met Vicki at the Providence Hospital annual new staff welcoming party a short time after she arrived in Denver. At Edward's suggestion, Alex also opened dialogue and eventually developed a working relationship, even friendship, with Vicki as he came to understand in his research that a support structure for coordination of physical and behavioral health was useless unless the doctors providing the care were willing to work together. Vicki had the knowledge and experience to make this happen. Her involvement and persuasion as a part of the innovation triumvirate was tantamount.

* * *

To recruit Dr. Vicki, Providence had demonstrated they were serious about correcting the poor psychiatric care provided on their general medical units, but to embark on the extensive and expensive reorganization met tremendous resistance.

Flatly, Providence balked at the financial impediments. The programs that Dr. Vicki recommended could necessitate supplemental funding from other clinical programs and a reduction in the already tenuous profit margin in order for mental health and substance-use specialists to make a decent living. Providence executives were sure that on a systemwide basis it would not fly. The hospital system and nonpsychiatrist physicians were not ready for it, and Vicki's program, though valuable, would cost money. Providence put on the brakes.

They said yes to an integrated care unit and a few psychiatric consultants at Providence General Hospital, yes to an additional behavioral health consultant team to provide psychiatric support in their seven other hospitals in Denver and the surrounding region, and yes to a nurse care manager or two in one or two of their multispecialty medical clinics. To go beyond would realize profits for health plans and purchasers, not for providers unless payment processes were changed. Why would they be willing to run a deficit to make health plans and businesses rich?

Early in her research on integrated programs, Vicki had puzzled over the self-same dilemma. Is equitable payment to clinicians and facilities for integrated care necessary before the integrated clinics and hospital programs are created, or is it the other way around? Health plans steadfastly refused to pay for integrated care until it had been proved effective. "Where's the supporting data?" they would ask. Likewise, clinical programs refused to develop them until they were equitably reimbursed. At first glance it appeared a stalemate, but deeper investigation proved otherwise.

To shatter the erroneous notion that providers would be the big losers, Vicki campaigned hard. With an educational blitz, she created a ruckus with Providence executives and its physicians, inundating them with information about the consequences of fragmented physical health and psychiatric care, the value of integration, and the steps needed to correct the problem in the Providence system.

Alex and Edward tirelessly met the challenge of persuading purchasers and health plan communities of the value in moving toward integrated care with their own educational blitz to businesses in the Denver region. They targeted moderate to large employers, such as Qwest, Northern States Power, EchoStar, and

Lockheed Martin. Because general assistance patients would undoubtedly be affected by the integrated system, they held discussions with leaders in the Colorado Department of Human Services and the Department of Health. Medicare and Medicaid program representatives also were brought up to speed on the health care integration issue. Discussions with these groups inevitably centered on state and federal bureaucracy roadblocks.

Alex used his influence as the president-elect of the Colorado Coalition of Businesses to spread the word among the business community. Many of his colleagues asked questions and challenged him because they still carved out their behavioral health to independent vendors, such as Ferdinand Behavioral (FB) and BVD. Their mindset remained congruent with the concept that mental health and substance-use disorder treatment should be separated from the rest of medicine and limited to the few "crazies" that caused society the most trouble.

The majority of businesses, aligned on dispensing health care, agreed that *no* money should be spent to treat people who abuse alcohol or drugs, as if this were different from the treatment of people who smoke or eat too much. Though lung cancer, emphysema, and diabetes could be just as much the result of poor impulse control as alcohol and drug abuse, few made the connection. To this large population of skeptics, Alex's message was a hard sell.

After several months of meetings and numerous fact-sharing presentations to large businesses, moderate- to small-sized business coalitions, and government agencies, they found that there was tremendous interest but little optimism about the likelihood of real change. Everyone was intrigued by the concept and saw the value that integrated care could bring. They were dubious about the promised return on investment. Instead, they remained fixated on other pressing issues directly related to short-term health care costs, such as medication benefit management, tiering of clinical practices, paying for provider performance, managing health plan administrative costs, pushing for improved case and disease management, and so on. For many, integrating physical and behavioral health had not yet hit their radar screens.

Faced with a doubting Thomas at every turn, Alex, Edward, and Vicki never surrendered to the pessimism. Strong behind-the-scene support fueled their resolve. Mr. Kishi, Alex's boss, had personal experience with the ineffectual, fragmented health care system, and Edward's boss at Ecumenical Care, Mr. Romani, was firmly in favor of promoting the greater good with quality products. The two men had arrived at their stations in life because they championed innovative ideas and failure was in neither man's vocabulary.

Mr. Romani, deeply invested in the public good, perhaps, a by-product of his religious upbringing, was well connected in the health industry and elevated the efforts of risk takers in the health plan community. He had a Midas touch, and with a market share to protect, onlookers at the other health plans kept a steady eye on his maneuvers. Further, he had learned that a small health plan in the Northwest had documented a 1.8 percent return on investment in the first year after instituting integrated case management for its members and 8.1 percent in the second. He was sure that the alliance that Edward had developed could do at least as well.

By winter of their first year of partnership, Alex, Edward, and Vicki knew their long suits and where they could be applied to achieve the ultimate goal of integrated health care. They also knew that in order to avoid dire financial implications both for providers and for health plans that both groups would have to make the transition simultaneously, almost in lockstep. Further, they would need strong purchasing partners.

THE ALLIANCE

Meeting regularly, the partners formulated several basic principals:

- Mental health and substance-use disorder care would become a clinical and administrative part of the basic benefit set at the clinical and health plan levels. Purchasers would buy one uniformly managed product, which always included behavioral health, no exclusions.
- Integrated care largely would take place in the primary care setting where the majority of psychiatric patients are seen. Medical access in psychiatric clinics and inpatient settings for patients with severe and persistent mental illness also would be a priority because poor outcomes were as common in this group.
- Patients at high risk for adverse outcomes due to combined physical and psychiatric illness would be identified proactively. Preventive measures would be employed, when possible, to reduce unnecessary or high-cost service use. The public health, not the social service, model would be adopted.
- Both physical and behavioral health specialists would be accountable for total health outcomes, not just those associated with their independent disciplines.
- Integrated clinical programs would enhance and/or complement independent physical health and mental health/substance-use disorder service delivery.
- All personal health information would be stringently protected from nonclinician access; however, physical and behavioral health information would be available to all clinicians caring for patients with concurrent physical and behavioral health problems, regardless of clinical discipline.

PROVIDER FACTOR

The Providence hospitals and clinics served the needs of a substantial percentage of ECI and Telstar employees. Approximately 40 percent of Ecumenical Care members used the Providence system, thus most Providence doctors were in Ecumenical Care's networks. This worked to Vicki's advantage in furthering her cause, as it did the Providence Health System's chief executive officer, Mr. Cooper. Embroiled in several high-exposure adverse-outcome lawsuits with the Providence system as defendant, he was open to any suggestion that would stop the bad publicity.

At Mr. Cooper's request, Vicki gave presentations to the hospitals' administrative leadership, to the physical health staff, and to mental health and substance-use disorder staff systemwide, documenting the interaction of physical and psychiatric illness, its effect on patients' clinical outcomes, and the relation to total cost of care. During the presentations, she outlined the specifics of the plan she had proposed to Mr. Cooper for creating an Integrated Physical and Behavioral Health Center of Excellence before accepting the position. With Mr. Cooper in attendance at many of the major presentations, he listened to the concerns discussed and lent legitimacy to Vicki's statements.

She explained that components of the initiative during the first four years included the introduction of a proactive case-finding instrument to identify complex patients, three multispecialty clinics supported by on-site mental health teams, and a coordinated and systemwide inpatient psychiatry consultation and emergency room service with 24-hour availability. There would be inpatient integrated care (medical psychiatry) units in the three largest hospitals in the system with staggered opening dates.[2] Last, a centralized psychiatric emergency capability at Providence General, the Providence system's largest and most centrally located hospital, would eventually be established.

Ancillary elements of the plan would include medical consultants assigned to cover physical health needs on stand-alone psychiatric units, emergency room mental health and substance-use disorder coverage at the other Providence general hospitals, and part-time mental health and substance-use disorder personnel to support dually trained care managers in other general medical clinics. One additional feature was the integration of the general medical and psychiatric electronic medical records system.

Concrete steps needed to implement the project with a three-year rollout included:

- Recruiting psychiatrists who specialized in the treatment of the medically ill (psychiatrists for the medically ill, or PMIs) to organize inpatient hospital and emergency room coverage.
- Developing mental health/substance-use disorder teams to support mental health care in the three multispecialty clinics.
- Adding and/or training existing nurse care managers to support both physical and behavioral health patient needs in other Providence clinics.
- Identifying an internist interested in serving as a consultant to the psychiatric clinics and inpatient units.
- Delineating clinical triggers for high-risk patients and implementation of a complex case-finding tool.
- Scheduling and training staff in integrated care.
- Identifying locations and renovations needed for the integrated care units in Providence General (general integrated unit), Providence St. Ignatius (pediatric integrated unit), and Providence Baptist (geriatric integrated unit) Hospitals and the psychiatric emergency room facilities at Providence General.
- Drawing architectural plans for the integrated care unit in Providence General.
- Sketching the communication and privacy rules for the integrated electronic medical record.

Development of the Providence General Hospital unit, the three integrated multispecialty clinics, inpatient psychiatric consultation services, and access to mental health and substance-use disorder support in the Providence emergency rooms would occur first. Designing the two other integrated care units and the regional centralized psychiatric emergency facility would take place in years three and four.

On the recommendation of Mr. Cooper, Providence Health System voted and the initial phase of Vicki's Integrated Physical and Behavioral Health Center of Excellence was accepted by a slim margin. It was show time.

PREPARING FOR INTEGRATED SERVICE DELIVERY

Annual contracts with the health plans were signed in early December with start dates of January 1. The announcement that Ecumenical Care would be partnering with the Providence Hospital system to help them develop the Integrated Center of Excellence gave incentive to employees to choose Ecumenical Care over other plans. Their market share increased 3 percent, whereas Medical Mart lost 2 percent of its market share—a significant hit given a starting base of only 18 percent.

By March, Dr. Mac, the head of family medicine and outpatient clinic director, was collaborating with Dr. James, a psychiatrist from a stand-alone psychiatric outpatient clinic who had always been interested in integrated care. Dr. Allen, a behavioral medicine–trained PhD psychologist, and Alice, a physical health clinical nurse specialist who wished to expand mental health and substance-use disorder capabilities in the Providence medical clinics, collaborated with Drs. Mac and James. Physical and behavioral health care managers were then woven into the multispecialty clinic's operations.

By May, this team was well along its way in setting up the clinical reorganization and work flows needed to transform the three multispecialty clinics so that assessing and addressing mental health and substance-use disorder issues were a standard part of clinic activity. All staff, not just the behavioral specialists, contributed to the decision-making process. The necessary work flow changes upset some staff, but those unwilling to adapt would move on.

An internist, Dr. Mason, had raised an autistic child and had a special interest in and understanding of patients with mental illness. He became the designate for physical health care for patients primarily seen in the psychiatry outpatient clinics. Shocked that so few were receiving preventive medical evaluations or routine follow-up care, he began with two half-days a week but increased the workload to three full days by the end of the year.

Vicki hired Dr. Kevin, a respected PMI in Denver, to run the psychiatric consultation program for Providence General. By June, he, two other psychiatrists, and two psychiatric clinical nurse specialists working as members of his consultation team were listed as members of the medical provider network for Ecumenical Care, the Blues, and two other health plans in Colorado, including Medical Mart.

This turn of events pleased FB because it would not be financially liable for the care given, but Medical Mart balked. Alex watched the drama at Medical Mart closely. He, however, did not know that internal discussions to drop the FB contract, unbeknownst to FB, were ongoing. Medical Mart could not afford to lose more market share. Members of its sales staff already were worried about next year. Even long-term customers threatened to find a new health plan unless Medical Mart did something, and soon.

As these changes got under way, one of the biggest challenges was resolving the privacy debate about what clinical information could be accessed and by whom. At first, the Health Insurance Portability and Accountability Act (HIPAA) and Colorado laws were used as excuses to restrict mental health/substance-use disorder information from being viewed by physical health clinicians. When no law could be found that prohibited clinicians involved in a patient's care from seeing both physical and behavioral health information in the Providence system, personal challenges surfaced.

Selected mental health and substance-use disorder professionals considered information they gathered too sensitive for the eyes and ears of physical health practitioners. Family physicians and general internists recoiled that the information they recorded was also sensitive—such as abortions, sexually transmitted diseases, alcohol withdrawal, drug overdoses, and so forth. They argued that all medical records should be protected from nonclinician access; however, to restrict communication between mental health, substance-use disorder, and physical health practitioners who treat the same patient would result in poor care. Clinicians in each area would be making important decisions that affected their patients lives, but without all the facts.

The opinion that all clinicians should have access to all pertinent clinical information and should have few roadblocks, with limited exceptions, prevailed. Firewalls in ECI's electronic medical records were opened to practitioners throughout the Providence system. Coordinated and collaborative communication between clinicians opened to provide integrated physical and behavioral health records by rollout of several of the integrated clinical programs. At the same time, state-of-the-art safeguards from unauthorized access also were given the highest priority.

Finally, after much wrangling about physical space in the medical setting, the Facilities Planning Committee at Providence General decided that Four Southeast, an old surgical unit surrounded by other medical units, would begin renovation in July to serve as the integrated care unit. The committee had wanted to put the unit across the street from the main general hospital because that location had unused space, but Vicki would have none of it. She pointed out that there were five major reasons that integrated care units closed within two to five years of their inception:

1. Beds were licensed as psychiatric, not medical; thus units quickly became financially insolvent with the limited per diems of the behavioral health system if physically sick patients, needing tests, consultations, and procedures, were admitted.

2. Nursing staff were not trained to provide both high-acuity physical health and psychiatric care, consequently targeted sick patients for integrated care, the ones most likely to benefit, were appropriately refused admission by nursing staff for safety reasons.

3. Physician coverage from either medicine or psychiatry was marginal, thus physicians would not refer their sick patients because of concern about quality-of-care issues.

4. Ownership and active involvement in unit development and operation was primarily psychiatric, with tacit internal medicine and/or family medicine sign-off; thus high-volume patient referrals from the physical health setting were not forthcoming.

5. The unit was located more than a five-minute walk or in another building from other medical units, thereby restricting nonpsychiatrist physician interest in admitting patients because of the difficulty in seeing patients easily on rounds. Getting timely medical tests and consultations completed and rapid response to emergency situations, such as cardiac arrests, also were impeded.

Vicki said she would rather put the initial unit in another Providence hospital than create a unit in the wrong location that was doomed to failure even before it opened. At Vicki's bidding, Mr. Cooper instructed the Facilities Planning Committee to find a medically accessible location in the main building of Providence General. If they were going to have a integrated care unit, why not put it where the sickest and most indigent patients were, thereby capturing cost-saving and length-of-stay-reducing (bed opening) benefits that occurred in the unit Vicki previously had run. She had found that an average of 350 admissions of the most complex patients per year to the medical psychiatry unit was associated with a $1.75 million savings compared to traditional care. Much of this savings was captured through reduced lengths of stay, an average of 1,400 bed-days. Because most admissions at Providence General were paid based on diagnostic related groups (DRG) rates or were indigent, the savings were tangible at the bottom line.

The aggressive movement toward integration was made easier because Mr. Cooper had received confirmation from Mr. Romani that the Ecumenical Care Foundation would kick in $500,000 over three years to support the development of the integrated program within the Providence health system. After Vicki's meeting with Ecumenical Care in December, Mr. Romani told his information systems division that he wanted to see whether a retrospective analysis of Ecumenical Care enrollees would yield the same results that Vicki had described.

Within two weeks, Vicki's prediction regarding the prevalence of cost shifting was confirmed (Figure 7.1). Medical service use for patients with mental health and substance-use disorders was massive compared to those without mental disorders. Further, patients who received a behavioral health diagnosis, but no apparent treatment, used as many health care services as those who received treatment. Treated patients, however, at least had the potential to get better, though prior studies now demonstrated that cost offset usually occurred in the second year.[3] Obviously, integrated care was advantageous.

Figure 7.1 Per-member-per-year claims expenditures for Ecumenical Care members with mental health diagnoses with and without mental health service use.
Telstar was able to confirm through claims data analyses that employees and family insured by Ecumenical Care who had mental health and substance-use disorders used more than twice the number of services as those without those disorders. Interestingly, nearly 40 percent of those with mental health or substance-use disorder problems had no recorded treatment for them in the claims records.

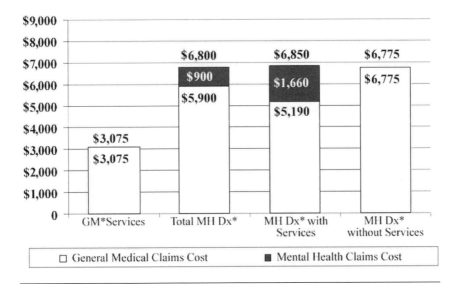

Mr. Romani also persuaded the Blues to match his contribution from their foundation. RockiesHealth, another health plan in Colorado that catered to Medicaid and Medicare recipients and had a vested interest in the value that integration brought to their patients, also matched Ecumenical Care's contribution. With pressure from FB to renew contract arrangements, Medical Mart was still on the fence, but with their market share already in jeopardy it would be only a matter of time before they took action.

Proactive Case Finding

A major addition to Vicki's integrated care organizational structure was a general medicine-based proactive case-finding instrument. Unlike in most medical settings where referrals are often made in reaction to incorrectly perceived mental health or substance-use disorder problems, Vicki chose ProAct to screen patients. The instrument had been developed and tested by a group of dedicated internists and psychiatrists in the medical setting to identify patients who would have the greatest likelihood of benefiting from integrated care.[4] It was short, easy to interpret, practical, and could be given by medical nursing staff or care managers.

ProAct was a computerized interdisciplinary complex-patient intervention guidance tool, which could be used in both the inpatient and outpatient settings. ECI assured Vicki and the information technology department at the Providence system that it could incorporate the tool as it installed their software. Every hospital admission could have an assessment if they exhibited identifiers, or red flags, for complexity, such as frequent clinic visits, many doctors, numerous medications, treatment nonresponse, high no-show rates, active or past history of psychiatric illness, and so forth.[5]

ProAct assessed historical, current state, and prognostic issues in the biological, psychological, social, and health system domains to determine which areas might require intervention for patients' health to improve. It focused on clinically relevant factors essential to treat patients successfully. For instance, blood pressure is the logical parameter to use to measure response to treatment for an elderly patient with hypertension. When blood pressure does not change after a proved antihypertensive medication is prescribed, then higher doses, other antihypertensives, or augmenting medications could be tried until control is accomplished (biological domain). Often, however, escalation of dose and increases in the number of medications does not result in persistent control, suggesting to the physician that the patient has treatment-resistant (refractory) hypertension.

Published reports suggest treatment resistance occurs in 50 percent or more of hypertensive patients. But can it actually be considered treatment-resistant if poor control can be reversed by providing assistance in domains other than the biological? Using ProAct, questions related to the health system, social, and psychological domains may provide clues about other areas in which intervention could lead to blood pressure control.

Continuing with the example of antihypertensive medication nonresponse, ProAct questions also inquire about the patient's ability to pay for the medications, which would fall under the health system domain: Did the patient even fill the prescription? Within the social domain, family availability to help a patient adhere to medication regime would be addressed: Did the patient often forget to take his pills? The psychological domain would investigate whether depression or another psychiatric condition existed: Did depression hamper the patient's will to follow his low-salt diet, control his weight, do his exercises, or take his pills?

ProAct was chosen because it was easily scored using visual pattern recognition in each domain: green, no problems; yellow, watch but no action; orange, consider action or keep an eye on the patient; red, attention now. A predominance of orange or red on a patient's summary sheet would prompt integrated health team involvement, because a combination of social, psychological, biological, and health system issues likely contributed to the patient's treatment resistance.

Years ago, when general physicians had the time to assess and evaluate person factors along with illness factors, intervention guidance tools such at ProAct were not necessary. The doctor would be able to glean from a breezy conversation whether her patient was exercising regularly or feeling overwhelmed about past-due bills. Nowadays, in a health care system that is preoccupied with reducing costs by focusing almost exclusively on biometrics, a tool like ProAct forces recognition of and intervention for psychological, social, and health system factors.

Staff Training

Working in absolutely separate cultures, mental health/substance-use disorders and physical health professionals are accustomed to roasting one another. More often then not, the interaction between the two is concentrated on glib put-downs like how one dumped patients on the other or poking fun at the other for not being able to take care of something so simple as helping a person through a family crisis (mental health personnel about medical personnel) or prescribing an antireflux agent for heartburn (medical personnel about psychiatrists or psychiatric nurse practitioners).

As Vicki added participants to her leadership team, she stressed useful techniques to quell the antagonistic atmosphere. Discussions about the overlap of symptoms in the two disciplines, and the negative effect that the interaction had on outcomes if not addressed, formed the core of the information shared in the series of presentations given to both inpatient and outpatient staff. The inherent mistrust and unspoken concerns, such as job restructuring or loss, change in authority and/or responsibility, and working with people who "trashed their discipline," however, were also critical areas to address in team building efforts.

The trainers covered core components needed to integrate care in the physical health setting: management of stress, depression, substance-use disorders, anxiety, unexplained somatic complaints, and the basics of good care management. All of the physical health clinic personnel, including doctors, were expected to attend. The conferences on outpatient training were interactive, with plenty of clinic-based case examples and an emphasis on maximizing each patient's clinical response and returning them to premorbid function.

By the time the integrated care practices were ready to come online, the integrated physical and behavioral health components of ECI's electronic medical record were described and privacy rules reinforced. All knew that they would lose their job if they accessed clinical information on patients with whom they did not have a patient-professional relationship. They also were instructed in the use of ProAct. Doctors, nurses, social workers, and others were expected to act in response to findings requiring immanent or immediate attention. Several additional sessions were used to resolve expected resistance and to minimize duplication of effort.

By the completion of training, which took about three months of weekly noon meetings, the staff began to understand how behavioral health was a vital part of physical health care. It would take months before the mental health and substance-use disorder staff introduced into this new setting would be accepted as a part of the team, but the stage was set to do away with "we" versus "they" thinking.

Dr. Mason also participated in the outpatient staff-training program, offering suggestions on how psychiatric assessments for depression and somatization could be added to the other preventive-care procedures triggered by ProAct and an integrated medical records system. Preventive care for psychiatric clinic patients, in fact, was where he and Vicki had decided to center his initial efforts. He certainly would be available for consultation and/or to provide support to mental health staff and physicians regarding physical health problems, but preventing unnecessary medical illness was the area in which he thought that he initially could bring the greatest value and save the most money.

* * *

Drs. Kevin and Vicki gave medical grand rounds on integrated care to physicians and other staff in the Providence system. They explained what integrated care was and described its components in the Providence system, including the medical psychiatry unit that would open at Providence General before the end of the year. They explained plans for psychiatric emergency facilities and integrated outpatient services as well as available access to rapid inpatient consultations at Providence General, St. Ignatius, and Baptist. Later on, other Providence hospitals would incorporate the same. They also mentioned the planned pediatric child psychiatry unit and geriatric medical psychiatry unit scheduled for St. Ignatius and Baptist, respectively, as a part of phase two.

The majority of time, however, was spent instructing physical health staff, unit nurses, and physicians in the use of the internal medicine and family practice–sponsored ProAct, which would also become operational throughout the medicine and family practice departments later in the year. Internal medicine and family practice nurses and physicians were encouraged to use ProAct scores and/or complexity patterns to identify patients who would benefit from assistance from the psychiatric consultation team. Where possible, ProAct components replaced other nursing admission assessments.

Finally, Vicki developed the educational program for nurses and other staff who would work on the Providence General medical psychiatry unit. She worked closely with the head of internal medicine and psychiatry nursing in establishing training modules. Basically, nurses recruited who had a medical background would undergo a three-week psychiatric nursing refresher and spend three weeks working on the general psychiatry unit at Providence General. Those recruited with a psychiatry background would participate in a three-week physical health refresher and spend three weeks working on an internal medicine unit.

For the first three months after the unit opened, all shifts would be staffed with at least one nurse with expertise in physical health and one in psychiatric inpatient care. During recruitment, preference would be given to nurses with longer experience in their area of expertise, though enthusiasm by the applicant for providing holistic care to patients was also an important factor. Historically, filling staff slots for medical psychiatry units always had been easy. Because many nurses believed that treating the whole person was a far better approach than treating either a physical or a behavioral illness in isolation, they welcomed the challenge and were eager to put in applications.

Integrating Service Delivery

Consistent with the challenge put forth by the Institute of Medicine Chasm Report, Vicki always stressed that patients were to be the center of the effort in all the various components of the integrated programs at Providence. If the clinical services they created did not lead to symptom alleviation and/or resolution and return the patient to maximum function, then the service was not worth constructing.

In addition, Vicki emphasized communication and collaboration between program components themselves and with the nonintegrated physical health and mental health/substance-use disorder settings. The formally integrated programs, which constituted the Integrated Center of Excellence, would provide a springboard for the education of general medical staff throughout the Providence system on how they could better address mental health and substance-use disorders in their clinical practices even when behavioral health specialists were not in the geographic area.

Integrated care was not something possible only in special programs; it was an integral part of physical health and psychiatric practice. Just too few mental health and substance-use disorder specialists were available to take care of the large number of patients with concurrent physical and behavioral illness. Plus, general medical practitioners had a leg up because they often already had an established relationship with their patients, the first step needed to set patients on the road to participating in their own health improvement.

Emergency Room Psychiatry and Behavioral Health Consultation

Only about 6 percent of emergency room visits have a component that is related to behavioral health, however, the number of patients who present with behavioral health problems has increased by 38 percent between 1992 and 2001, compared to an 8 percent overall increase for emergency rooms during the same period. Notably, substance-use disorder issues are four times as likely to use emergency rooms.[6] As well, Colorado, along with a least 35 other states, has a shortage of psychiatric beds.[7] Suicidal, psychotic, manic, and severely anorexic patients can wait in emergency rooms for days or be sent by ambulance to other hospitals, as was documented in a recent survey reported by Glenn Howatt in the *Minneapolis Star Tribune* (Figure 7.2), sometimes literally hundreds of miles away, to a facility with an open psychiatric bed. Alternatively, they may be admitted to a physical health unit, receive little if any psychiatric care during their stay, and end up creating medico-legal risks similar to the suicide by toilet paper on the medicine unit, which led to the Providence system's lawsuits.

The initial program that Vicki devised for Providence was to transform a portion of each emergency room to allow safe assessment and observation of patients with psychiatric issues. Existing general medical emergency room physicians, nurses, and social workers would be updated on how to deal with common psychiatric

**Figure 7.2 Minneapolis hospital-to-hospital transfers of mentally ill patients.
Glen Howatt at the *Minneapolis Star Tribune* documents what happens to patients presenting for emergency room services in Minnesota, where a shortage of psychiatric beds
is a major problem.**

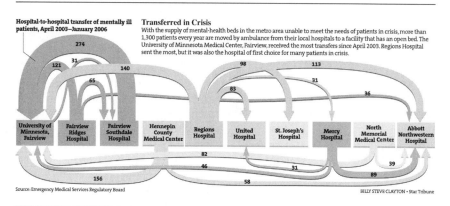

Source: "Transferred in Crisis" from an article entitled "No Room Here," *Minneapolis Star Tribune,* April 23, 2006.
Reprinted with permission from the *Minneapolis Star Tribune.*

presentations in the emergency room while they waited for assistance from members of the psychiatry consultation service who would maintain a 24-hour call
system. A selected set of nurses at each site, and in a floating pool, would be
trained to supervise the care of patients who needed psychiatric admission or at
least assistance with psychiatric illness in the general medical setting but were
awaiting a bed.

At some hospitals with a high emergency room throughput, such as Providence
General, one or two psychiatric emergency room staff, psychiatrists and nurses,
would be added to or replace existing personnel, especially during peak hours.
Every attempt would be made to keep a few psychiatric beds open in the Providence system at the end of each day in the event that an emergency admission
occurred. Again, with the bed shortages, this was not always possible.

The longer-term emergency room solution involved the development of a citywide psychiatric emergency facility to which police, ambulances, and community
agencies could bring or send patients. Because more than 40 percent of emergency room patients with psychiatric needs are not insured, no hospital clamored
to offer the service. In the long run, however, consolidating emergency care made
sense from safety and efficiency standpoints. Because Vicki had introduced the
concept, a number of agencies, government programs, and hospitals were discussing the pros and cons of public and private funding for a centralized psychiatric
emergency service, which potentially could prevent costly disasters, both in terms
of life and property.

To address the clinical situation once patients with mental health and substance-
use disorders got into the inpatient physical health setting, what Vicki put together

had several distinguishing characteristics. First, ProAct would inform referrals to mental health consultation teams. Projections, based on this instrument, indicate that the percentage of patients referred with illness who would benefit from psychiatric involvement would increase from 40 percent to 80 percent or more. In the current system, not only were few referred, but 60 percent of those referred had problems that easily could have been handled by support from their general physical health physicians and/or nursing staff.

Second, ProAct would increase the number of patients referred early in their general medical hospitalization. Outcome data on inpatient psychiatric consultation services clearly showed that patient referrals during the last 24 hours of hospitalization, which is the current standard, added to cost without providing lasting benefit to patients.

Third, Vicki stationed mental health teams at each hospital. Nurse clinicians, social workers, behavioral medicine–trained psychologists, and PMIs working as a coordinated group replaced the standard isolated psychiatrist or nurse clinician. Because general medical hospital stays were too short to warrant involvement of formal psychotherapists, team members became the conduits through which patients gained access to psychotherapy practitioners in a mental health sector that continued to provide specialized services.

Finally, under the supervision of a PMI, mental health and substance-use disorder teams extended the reach and contribution behavioral health makes to their physical health colleagues. More patients could be seen at lower cost and with regular follow-ups. Psychiatric consultations would move from a crisis-intervention orientation to an integral component necessary for outcome change as the programs matured.

INTEGRATED INPATIENT CARE

Treating the most severely ill with active physical and psychiatric illness in an inpatient medical psychiatry unit was Vicki's professional mission. The units she envisioned at Providence were similar in clinical capabilities to the one she had run for more than ten years at a university hospital in another state before taking the job in Denver. Because only a small fraction of the 30 percent with psychiatric comorbidity in the medical setting would be sufficiently ill to warrant the specialized care possible in the inpatient integrated setting, it was important that the medical psychiatry unit complement and support consultation and emergency room services.

Vicki had been in contact with many who wished to start medical psychiatry units and many others who already were running units. A survey she had instigated several years before documented that there was a large variance in the organization and capabilities of existing units. Based on studies and her own experience in taking care of patients with high-acuity concurrent general medical and psychiatric illness, she decided to open three units within the

Providence system. Despite different target populations, they would have the following common characteristics:

- Target severely ill complex patients with concurrent physical and psychiatric illness.
- Initiate evidence-based and coordinated physical and psychiatric treatment on the first day of hospitalization in a safe environment by staff with the training to do so.
- Complement and enhance care on existing general medical and psychiatric units and collaborate with medical and psychiatric consultation services that would care for less severe and/or complex patients in the physical health and psychiatric settings.
- Maximize clinical, financial, and functional outcomes.

As well, in line with a core set of operational guidelines (Table 7.1), Vicki adapted inpatient settings that allowed customization of services that would meet the needs of target populations, such as children/adolescents and the elderly. She intended to put a pediatric psychiatry unit in St. Ignatius, the Providence system's children's hospital, and a geriatric medical psychiatry unit in Baptist, located in an older section of town with a large population of elderly and frail patients.

Between March and June, the hospital architects made several revisions of floor plans to transform Four Southeast (a 26-bed surgical unit already scheduled for renovation) into a 10-bed medical unit and a 12-bed locked medical psychiatry unit. They would lose four beds as a result of the transition due to psychiatric safety and program requirements. Even with the bed reduction, as a result of shortened lengths of stay for complex patients admitted to this more efficient clinical setting, they anticipated greater bed capacity for patient admissions.

The medical psychiatry unit would have the same physical health care capabilities found on other general medical units and psychiatric capabilities as on the acute general psychiatry unit at Providence General. Central lines, peritoneal dialysis, infectious isolation procedures, and respiratory therapy would

---

Table 7.1
Core Medical Psychiatry Unit Organizational Guidelines

- Collaboratively administered and staffed by a general medical physician and a psychiatrist for the medically ill or by a physician jointly trained in internal medicine and psychiatry
- Identification and renovation of clinical space contiguous with other general or specialty medical units in the general hospital with physical characteristics that meet state and federal licensure and safety requirements for both physical health and psychiatric care
- Training in cross-disciplinary work processes for all nursing and social service unit staff directed by internal medicine and psychiatry nursing departments
- Consolidation of general medical and psychiatric policies and procedures to accommodate patients with concurrent illness
- Nurse and physician staffing patterns, physical space design, and policies and procedures that are capable of safely addressing the needs of the most severely impaired patients to be admitted

---

Note: Organizational guidelines for inclusion of outcome-changing components in the development of a medical psychiatry unit.

be just as available as rapid use of medication to control hallucinations and delusions (rapid neuroleptization). Around-the-clock supervision for suicidal patients, behavior modification for emaciated eating-disorder patients, and electroconvulsive therapy for manic or suicidally depressed patients also would be provided.

* * *

The decision to locate the unit had been made in March. At this point, it was possible to develop a timeline for project completion. Mr. Cooper had put unit renovation on the fast track, which had been part of the agreement with the Ecumenical Care Foundation.

- March to June: Develop physical space architectural design.
  - *Psychiatric features:* Locked entrance; dining and day room; seclusion room; mostly single rooms; laundry facilities, refreshment room; water shutoff valves; wireless telephones, storage area for patient belongings; video surveillance capabilities in most patient rooms, shatterproof glass and mirrors; hang-proof closet, curtain, shower rods, plumbing fixtures, and doorknobs; shortable electric sockets; barricade-proof doors and durable furniture; no long cords; tamperproof lights and ceiling; sharps containers in the nursing station.
  - *Medical features:* Medical gases, private bathrooms, wide doors for bed passage, physical examination room, clean and dirty utility rooms, equipment storage room, infectious isolation room, cardiac arrest cart, janitorial service room and linen closet, bathtub room.
- April and May: Recruit and hire medical psychiatry unit head nurse and social worker.
- May through September: Rewrite medical and psychiatric policies and procedures to accommodate patients with concurrent illness (extensive and time-consuming), establish staffing and work flows.
- June and July: Send out bid requests for renovation to contractors; purchase renovation materials and equipment.
- June through August: Recruit integrated care unit nursing staff (including specialized floating staff); establish necessary links and services (e.g., activity therapy, occupational therapy, electroconvulsive therapy, pharmacy, etc.).
- August to October: Physical space renovation; observe and troubleshoot process.
- August and September: Train medical psychiatry unit nursing staff; establish physician and resident coverage for both internal medicine and psychiatry; advertise unit opening in October with a media blitz about and presentations on the Integrated Physical and Behavioral Health Center of Excellence opening in the Providence Hospital system.
- October 1 to October 15: Staff orientation.
- October 15: Open unit with six beds.
- October 15 to December 15: Ramp up to 12 beds; adjust and adapt work processes, policies and procedures, staffing and coverage patterns to accommodate patients and providers served.

INTEGRATED OUTPATIENT CARE

Psychiatric services in the three multispecialty medical clinics were organized so that as many complex patients as possible could receive the treatment they needed in order to alleviate both their physical health and psychiatric symptoms. This would start by sharing information with internists and family physicians about the relationship between high medical service use, poor medical illness control, and the presence of psychiatric symptoms. They would receive training in ProAct, the value it brought to patient care, and how to use it.

ProAct screening in previously identified at-risk patients would be the clue for primary and specialty physical health physicians about which patients were complex and which health domains needed attention and how swiftly. Conservative testing and intervention for unexplained somatic complaints would be possible because the physical health doctors would be trained in how to protect patients from unnecessary tests and medications.

As important, those with concurrent psychiatric problems would be aggressively treated, with the help of the imbedded mental health team if necessary, and close attention would be paid to physical and mental health/substance-use disorder treatment adherence. As with so many new initiatives, use of ProAct would require restructuring clinic work flows to make sure that patients with orange and red markers on ProAct summary sheets received appropriate attention.

Because the integration project was a collaborative effort between the Blues, Ecumenical Care, and RockiesHealth, physicians in the Providence system would have greater access to care management services available through each of these health plans. Further, there was every indication that many other health plans would come on board during the coming year.

Vicki considered ProAct and physician training necessary, but not sufficient, to change outcomes for patients with concurrent physical and behavioral problems or medical manifestations of psychiatric illness. In order to realize the goal of a fully integrated program, the on-site health professionals, who could serve as care managers under the direction of a PMI, was the linchpin to success.

To this end Dr. Mac, Dr. James, Dr. Allen, and Alice were actively involved in the process of setting up integrated care for the three multispecialty clinics. Each clinic had slightly different needs based on the population that it served. Denver Metropolitan Clinic, located across the street from St. Ignatius Children's Hospital, supported a large pediatric practice. In this clinic, they would develop an integrated pediatric, child psychiatry, and child psychology program. Another clinic was located adjacent to a retirement village near Baptist Hospital. Here, they would create an integrated geriatric program with affiliations to several nursing homes in the surrounding neighborhood. In addition, they would add an integrated component in the family and general medicine clinics that served nearby ECI.

The last clinic, adjacent to Providence General, served a large percentage of patients in public programs, such as Medicaid, medical assistance, and Medicare. This location would be integrated and serve as the primary care clinic with special behavioral health capabilities, such as a buprenorphine or methadone-maintenance

Table 7.2
Core Integrated Clinic Organizational Guidelines

Administration
Administered by general medicine department with a psychiatrist as part of the clinical team (pediatrician and child psychiatrist in the case of St. Ignatius)

Location
Collocation of behavioral health, care management, and general medical staff within a general medical clinic

Organizational system
Proactive behavioral health assessments for patients with orange (many) or red (all) flags on the ProAct and physician training in working with unexplained physical complaints

Work processes
- Nearly immediate access for primary care physicians and their patients to a behaviorally trained nurse or social service case manager supervised by a psychiatrist
- Same-day appointments
- Regular communication among clinic staff; case management involvement based on ProAct-determined complexity

Communication
Close interaction and reciprocal arrangements with the external mental health system such as off-site full-service mental health programs and substance-use disorder clinic staff with capabilities for formal psychotherapy, intensive partial programs, substance use disorder treatment, and so forth

Note: Core features required to assure clinical improvement and maximize resource utilization in patients when setting up a general medical clinic with mental health and substance-use disorder access and capabilities.

clinic for opium addicts and integrated substance-use disorder program for patients with alcohol dependence complicated by medical issues. All clinics would use core integrated clinic organizational guidelines (Table 7.2).

No one expected the development of the integrated clinics to be easy, because it involved cultural reorientation and new work processes for both physical and behavioral health staff. Vicki's experience, however, had been positive with regard to recruiting, training, and retention. Nursing staff in properly formulated integrated care clinics took great pride in what they did. Once trained, they stuck around and developed a new culture that led to helping the whole patient, rather than just an illness or an isolated problem.

Then there was the challenge of recruiting professionals from shortage disciplines, such as psychiatry and child psychiatry.[8] Because a triple board residency program was already in place in Denver (pediatrics, psychiatry, child psychiatry), Vicki was hopeful that they would be able to attract a couple of jointly trained pediatrician-child psychiatrists. She also was in contact with directors of a number of the 17 internal medicine and psychiatry and 11 family practice and psychiatry residency programs, which were fertile ground for recruitment.

To have the integrated multidisciplinary clinics operational before the integrated inpatient unit at Providence General opened in October and concurrent with the inpatient consultation services was the goal. It was a lofty goal and dependent on the interaction of the health plans and the purchasers who bought them.

Chapter 8

A NEW GENERATION
OF HEALTH CARE

If you can dream it, you can do it. Remember this whole thing was
started with a dream and a mouse.[1]

—Walt Disney

A NECESSARY PARTNERSHIP

As Vicki's integrated programs developed, health plans simultaneously transi-
tioned. In response to increased demand from purchasers for a more functional
integrated mental health and substance-use disorder product, Ecumenical Care's
decision to insource behavioral health had been made long before ECI and Telstar
took interest in revamping the health care system. The dedication to health care
integration was no less dramatic at Ecumenical Care than it was in the Providence
system.

Recognizing the need to do something creative to bring about change and well
attuned to the magnitude of the transition process, Mr. Romani had signed off on
internal restructuring at Ecumenical Care. Gut instinct assured him that in the
long run the up front costs and the staggering realignment process would pay off
in terms of health outcomes for members, profit, and customer care.

Importantly, the replacement health plan system for dealing with members having psychiatric illness (i.e., integrating behavioral and physical health business
practices) would be considerably less cumbersome and less costly than the current
carved-out or even carved-in system. He estimated that internal administrative
costs of claims adjudication alone would be a quarter to a third less when the
conversion was complete. Consolidation of documentation software, customer

and provider services, and care management practices also offered opportunities for cost savings. This would all occur internally while predicted returns would accumulate through reduced claims, especially in the second year. Savings would accrue to both Ecumenical Care through its fully insured customers and to its self-insured accounts.

Ecumenical Care, a not-for-profit company, had been a fringe player in the health plan market, picking up business mainly from provider-based health delivery operations in the region. They always had based their decisions about how they supported services as much on ethical and quality of care considerations as they had on profitability, and they had never shied away from introducing innovative products.

With a view toward the future, Mr. Romani knew that Ecumenical Care could not make the move toward integration alone. Other health plans in the area eventually would have to support integrated service as well for clinical programs outside of the Providence system to change the way they provided clinical care and for it to become available system-wide. As the trailblazer, he would be first in line to significantly increase Ecumenical Care's market share. If momentum was not maintained, Ecumenical Care also could slip into Colorado's health care history. For the good of Ecumenical Care enrollees, he decided to gamble.

Under Mr. Romani's direction and long before the contract with BVD expired, Ecumenical Care's contracting and benefits personnel met with Vicki, Mr. Cooper, and the Providence system's chief financial officer. Together they discussed general principles about health plan reimbursement considered necessary for the Integrated Physical and Behavioral Health Center of Excellence to work.

- Behavioral health specialists with billing capabilities would have to: (1) be credentialed as a part of the physical health network; (2) be listed in health plan publications with other physical health practitioners; (3) bill using similar coding procedures as physical health disciplines in whose clinics they now worked with similar co-pays, coinsurance, and treatment duration limits; and (4) be paid from now-combined physical and behavioral health benefits.

- Authorization and reporting procedures for behavioral health care and its practitioners needed to be comparable among all medical disciplines treating behavioral disorders.

- Reimbursement to all mental health and substance-use disorder clinicians for the treatment they provided should encourage them to work in the medical setting (i.e., adequate amounts, low hassle factor, etc.). Further, a mechanism to support personnel should be in place under the direct supervision of psychiatrists to extend their short supply, especially clinical nurse specialists and physician assistants.

- Physical health and mental health/substance-use disorder practitioners should be able to see and bill for discrete patients on the same day.

Mr. Romani worked alongside Edward as they developed stopgap measures, which would support the clinical environment that Vicki was creating in the Providence system. Mr. Cooper could not and would not make the changes necessary to effect altered outcome unless he could see that profitability would be the endgame. It was one thing to rectify problems that led to a lawsuit and another to put your hospital and clinic system in financial jeopardy while doing so. Mr. Romani was certain that the latter would not happen. In the long run, Mr. Romani saw this as a win-win situation for him and Mr. Cooper. If he created a reimbursement environment that supported integrated care, he would save money in both administrative and claims costs. He would save money internally and have a more competitive product to sell purchasers. Mr. Cooper would likewise profit as reimbursement practices became consistent and sufficient to cover costs and add profit to the clinical operations.

Edward and he started by creating work-arounds for the practitioners in the Providence integrated programs. These included:

- Reassigning the mental health and substance-use disorder inpatient consultants, those working in integrated outpatient settings, and medical psychiatry unit personnel, who used assessment and intervention practices approved by the health policy committee (e.g., here-and-now psychotherapies, appropriately dosed medications, etc.) to have billing privileges within the physical health physician network. Claims for patients treated by them would be paid from physical health benefits with equivalent co-pays and coinsurance using comparable medical coding and billing procedures. Both Mr. Romani and Edward reasoned that they were paying primary care physicians for these services already but with worse outcomes (Figure 7.1).

- Mental health and substance-use disorder licensed practitioners working in the medical setting who were not able to directly bill for services (e.g., social workers, master's level psychologists, registered psychiatric nurses, etc.) would be paid through physician-based supervisory arrangements.

- Mental health and substance-use disorder personnel could bill for services provided on the same day as physical health practitioners, whether in the inpatient or outpatient setting.

- Mental health and substance-use disorder prior authorization procedures in the integrated setting were suspended for the first five visits.

- No behavioral health diagnosis was required for the first three visits in order to be paid.

- On the medical psychiatry unit Vicki described, concurrent care authorization would not take place before the eighth day of hospitalization, with occasional exceptions. In selected patients, these concurrent reviews would be suspended altogether.

- Per-visit reimbursement rates for mental health and substance-use disorder personnel would be adjusted to a level slightly greater than that for comparable personnel performing similar tasks in the behavioral health setting. At least as a start, reduction in hassles and increased reimbursement for services should encourage a redistribution of psychiatric personnel from established practice settings.

With these work-arounds in place, allowing Mr. Cooper and Vicki to move forward with their clinical program development, the first order of business for

Edward and Mr. Romani was to constitute a transition task force composed of key members of each division at the health plan (Figure 6.1). The 15 members on the task force were professionals who knew the business of fund distribution. They were charged with the mission of reconfiguring Ecumenical Care's care support capabilities so that they would encourage integrated care throughout the region. Based on their skill sets, task force members set up networks, credentialed providers, wrote both provider and subscriber contacts, marketed and sold products, set policy for response to queries and complaints, created programs to manage and assist members through case management, and adjudicated claims.

Because mental health and substance-use disorders had never been a significant concern on the fund distribution level, early efforts focused on identifying stumbling blocks that they were bound to encounter. They held brainstorming seminars on integration, gathering insight and suggestions from frontline staff. Nevertheless, with work flows in flux, ever-present resistance instigated more problems than solutions.

Staffs in each of Ecumenical Care's divisions (i.e., sales and marketing, networking, contracting, customer service, claims, information systems, health management, actuary and finance, legal, and quality assurance) were expanded largely with professionals from mental health and substance-use disorder backgrounds. As they came on board, all were apprised of the core concepts of integrated physical and behavioral health and how it differed from insourced behavioral health (mental health and substance-use disorder staff "owned" by the medical managed care company without real integrated work flow and business process change).

To incite enthusiasm, Ecumenical Care employees wore lapel pins announcing "Concurrent Care, not Sequential Care." Though few outside the company understood the message, when asked, employees spoke out in one voice. "From the time of their initial visit, our members will get both physical health and psychiatric services, regardless of location."

By the first of January, regional mental health and substance-use disorder providers had been credentialed in the general medical network with behavioral health an integral part of the medical call-in system. The case and disease management staff expanded to include psychiatric nurses and social workers. If these individuals were not certified in case or disease management within three years, they would not be retained. Mental health and substance-use disorder staff in both customer service and care management were mixed in with existing physical health staff pods. Members of each pod helped cross-disciplinary coworkers address all individual client issues through the indirect assistance of other pod members.

Ecumenical Care's finance director and the claims processor worked closely with selected team members to create an integrated-care contracting and claims adjudication system. Another health plan in the western United States had introduced similar business process changes several years before and had experienced substantial reductions in service use by their Medicaid members (Table 8.1). Ecumenical Care actuaries were able to use this and internal data on their own risk pool to develop per-member-per-month amounts to charge for the new integrated care products. Based on the integrated service-saving data, purchasers who

Table 8.1
Western Integrated Care Management: Net Savings $400 per Member per Month

- 22% decrease in office visits
- 26% decrease in emergency room visits
- 72% decrease in hospital admissions
- 76% decrease in hospital days
- 24% decrease in medical services and pharmaceutical costs

Note: A health plan in the western United States documented a $400 savings per member per month by introducing health plan–level integration of physical and mental health/substance-use disorder support for Medicaid patients. These savings showed up as a reduction of total health care service use, presumably from the improved integrated treatment and clinical outcomes.

Source: Adapted from *Managed Healthcare Executive,* http://www.managedhealthcareexecutive.com/coloradoaccess.

wished to carve out behavioral health services actually would need to be charged more than those who purchased it in-house because the external behavioral health vendor merely would be cost-shifting the behavioral health service use to Ecumenical Care's general medical providers.

An added bonus was that in the new system there would no longer be the necessity of a separate adjudication process for mental health and substance-use disorder claims. Although this would need to be phased in over several years, by doing so they would eliminate up to a third of their behavioral health claims' processing costs, an activity for which they had paid BVD dearly. Finally, with a single claims system, it would be possible to track total health care costs for individual members and analyze component costs more readily.

The finance director and claims processor helped the contracting department create several integrated offerings of preferred provider organizations (PPOs), health maintenance organizations (HMOs), and consumer-driven health plans (CDHPs) for their clients. They also retained some old contracts, recognizing that these eventually would need to be phased out. The new contracts contained no mental health or substance-use disorder service opt-out conditions, nor were there differences in co-pays, coinsurance, or annual and lifetime limits between physical and behavioral health services. Not surprisingly, a revolutionary health plan like Ecumenical Care's that featured mental health and substance-use disorder benefits equal to physical health proved to be an easy sell in the Denver market.

Negotiating rates for provider contracts outside the Providence and University systems was not so easy. Though a majority of health care delivery systems recognized the need to bolster mental health and substance-use disorder support and were aware that many nonbehavioral specialists wanted greater access to psychiatric services, they resisted. Egos, pocketbooks, and facility solvency were at issue. The assorted providers, each wanting its piece of the pie, inspired lively jockeying among the different disciplines and between the hospital and clinic systems. The usual discussions about rates and discounts, practice tiering, formularies, pay for performance, and covered services reached a higher pitch.

Ecumenical Care's provider contract negotiators forced the issue of improving support for mental health and substance-use disorder services in discussions with physician groups, clinics, and hospital systems even if they competed with procedure-oriented and other programs that were already receiving top dollar. The target was to set equal net negotiated rates for all services. It would be the distribution of reimbursement to different professionals and clinical services that should change. Ecumenical Care negotiators were assured that with the increase in market share from industry contracts, such as Telstar and others, it was likely that provider groups would play ball. The prediction was accurate.

Over time, Ecumenical Care retained good contracted rates with most health systems in the area and picked up additional contracts along the way. With solid statistics backing improved care and the cost advantages of integration, Ecumenical Care was able to increase reimbursement to mental health and substance-use disorder practitioners and psychiatric service settings willing to integrate their services with their medical colleagues. As the integration concept caught on, more and more mental health and substance-use disorder practitioners chose to practice in the medical setting, which further increased interest in reimbursement parity.

Perhaps one of the most challenging components of Ecumenical Care's change to the internal integration of physical and behavioral health service support was configuring their information system to allow it to address physical health and psychiatric problems at the same time and in the same patients. Ecumenical Care's current software was not designed to perform both physical health and behavioral health medical necessity reviews or case and disease management, nor did it contain the ability for unimpeded communication.

Ruth, a psychiatric nurse certified in case management, and Jackie, a medical case manager, were set to the task of researching the software possibilities. Few vendors had products that met integrated care documentation needs, and transitioning to a user-friendly system was tedious and time-consuming. These operational matters, however, did not deter them. Along with their frontline staff, they developed work-arounds.

In anticipation of the need to develop a usable clinical documentation system, Ecumenical Care put out a request for proposal to several national case-management software vendors. Vying for first dibs on a product that was considered to have tremendous growth potential, at least three vendors submitted very reasonable bids. Ecumenical Care's utilization, case, and disease management staff chose the most promising from a large and stable vendor. They got an excellent bargain because they served as a beta test site for the software during the development phase.

Edward kept Mr. Romani abreast of progress both at Ecumenical Care and Providence. Mr. Romani cautioned Edward to make sure that contract benefit descriptions and Ecumenical Care's infrastructure encouraged and supported integrated clinical services in mental health and substance-use disorders, especially in the medical setting. If they were going to make these changes internally, it was exceedingly important that they led to an integrated clinical environment that changed patient outcomes. Edward, who attended most of the integration task force meetings as an interested bystander, confirmed that Ecumenical Care personnel kept this foremost in their minds.

On the cutting edge, Mr. Romani had set the pace and the standard for other health plans to follow. The transition to an insourced behavioral health business at Ecumenical, though tedious, had come about with few glitches. Sales and marketing, contracting and benefit design, and networking and credentialing had fallen into place. The internal mechanics of the change were a little more challenging, but legal, customer and provider service, health management, claims, information systems, finance, and quality improvement had made the transition with limited disruption in operations. They had realized a measurable increase in market share with promising opportunities ahead as integration mushroomed into the national arena.

SPREADING THE WORD

Nearly five years earlier, a couple of inconsistent tables in a slide presentation had inflamed Alex's curiosity. Ultimately, it enlightened a failing industry. The unlikely alliance of a human resources health care purchaser, a health plan vice president of operations, and an internist-psychiatrist had torched a campaign that yielded remarkable results. The combination of employer interest in the development of an integrated product, health plan responsiveness to employer interest, and an astute clinical system capable of initiating the project demonstrated the power of a collaborative effort.

Throughout the challenging process of building Providence's Integrated Physical and Behavioral Health Center of Excellence, Alex, Edward, and Vicki gave numerous presentations. Time and again, in one venue after another, they explained the enormous advantages of the integration project and the step-by-step approach to accomplishing it. The message ignited interest in other purchasers, health plans, hospitals, and clinics, and gradually integration became a buzzword in the industry.

Initially, it was Alex's regional business coalition and the university hospitals, then the Denver Chamber of Commerce, then a coalition of small business owners that spearheaded progress. By the end of the summer and into the fall, the Colorado Department of Human Services, the Department of Health, and the Department of Commerce had asked for information on how integrated care might impact Colorado state employees and those whose health care was supported by public programs funds.

In a small way, Alex, Vicki, and Edward had become celebrities. They were summoned to present at a national employer conference, the Quality and Best Practices Conference of the National Blues Association, and a national conference of the American Hospital Association. In every town, behind every podium, their message was simple:

- In the current fragmented system, many of the most complex and highest-cost patients had concurrent physical and behavioral health disorders, which were not being treated effectively.

- Service use (cost of care) in these patients was double or more and primarily came from costs associated with inadequately addressed mental health and substance-use disorder problems shifted to physical health benefit use for unnecessary visits, tests, and medications (80% or more of the health care dollar spent).
- Lack of treatment perpetuated the high-service-use cycle.
- Treatment of mental health and substance-use disorders using integrated physical health and mental health approaches in the medical setting was associated with a return toward health, resolution (or at least alleviation) of impairment, and reduced health care/disability costs.
- Changing this downward slide of health care was impossible when mental health and substance-use disorders were managed independently from physical health disorders.

The research supporting their points was robust and the saving potential substantial with early documentation. The message stuck. As a result of their presentations, more and more businesses in Colorado were asking their health plans about integrated products, which, in turn, kindled national interest. Many medical health plans already had insourced their mental health and substance-use disorder business. They also were investigating what it would take to move from insourced to integrated products. Those that had not insourced planned to do so during the next business cycle.

Most important, hospitals and multispecialty clinics, other than Providence, were now eager to set up integrated clinical programs. Administrative staff and clinicians alike recognized that integration would improve patient care while contributing to a profitable bottom line for hospitals, clinics, and, interestingly, health plans. Even purchasers benefited. More efficient health plan administration from consolidated physical and behavioral health business practices made premium reductions possible for both fully and self-insured plans. The greatest return, however, came from lower disability claims and greater employee productivity.

CLINIC FACTOR

Under Vicki's leadership, the integrated care unit at Providence General maintained 90 percent occupancy and regularly treated an array of patients, including suicidal depressed patients on dialysis; physically unstable patients withdrawing from drug and alcohol addictions; postsurgery psychotic and/or delirious patients; and self-mutilating patients. As a result of Dr. Kevin's delirium prevention program, the number of patients experiencing delirium was reduced by a third.

Without mishap, the Providence system had provided care for many psychiatrically dangerous and very physically sick patients. Most Four Southeast patients were discharged much more rapidly than they would have been in the old system. Physical and mental health treatment from day one was better than the old sequential model of treating first in general medicine, then discharge, and finally readmission to psychiatry for mental health treatment. Because Four Southeast unit procedures, physical organization, and nursing staff trained in concurrent care efficiently could reverse both the medical and psychiatric components of complex health problems, lengths of stay for Four Southeast patients were on average four days shorter than for comparable patients in other Providence hospitals. As well, when the Providence system expanded access to the Providence General unit by using the ProAct case identification process, patient transfers occurred rapidly from other hospitals within the system when beds were available on the integrated care unit.

The pediatric psychiatry and geriatric medical psychiatry units had opened with quality staff. With the upgrades in reimbursement for psychiatric care in the medical setting, these programs ran in the black—a boon that would have been impossible in the years before the integration initiative. Although start-up costs for the units were much greater than other components of Vicki's Integrated Physical and Behavioral Health Center of Excellence programs, the return on investment was much more rapid than the hospital expected. Even with the expanded capabilities of the pediatric and geriatric units, plans for new or renovated facilities in the Providence system always included consideration of additional integrated-care beds.

It took awhile for medical staff to get used to ProAct in both the inpatient and outpatient settings because physicians were initially reluctant to question the appropriateness of their earlier referral methods, much like the resistance P.C.A. Louis and Ignaz Semmelweis experienced in nineteenth century. Further, it required that staff address clinically relevant issues that previously had been ignored. Now forced to surmount social, psychological, and health system impediments to improve their patients, clinicians and their staff acknowledged the importance of supporting an intervention-focused case-finding system. Suggestions, clinically based rather than health plan–based, surfaced on how to improve clinical outcomes for patients and to reduce costs. This promoted several new ways in which health plans reimbursed for care and issued new legislation for patients covered by public programs. Positive-sum competition was taking root.

The first two years in which proactive psychiatric inpatient and emergency room consultation and outpatient integrated care practices were introduced were the most challenging. Because the system never had supported prevalence-based mental health and substance-use disorder intervention in the past, consolidating work practices and staffing levels that maximized benefits to patients took effort. On this front, ProAct definitely helped.

Personnel and their understanding of psychiatric care in the outpatient medical setting played a large role in measuring the success of each program. Because they had to be accessible to the primary and specialty physical health clinicians and their patients, behavioral health practitioners in integrated clinics could not fill their days doing therapy. They also had to be result-oriented, like their physical health colleagues, and yet retain the ability to build relationships with patients while moving them toward symptom and functional improvement.

Much activity in supplying psychiatric service to patients with physical illnesses related to educating patients, assisting them with physical health-support activities, following them for both physical and behavioral health treatment adherence, and documenting progress. Appropriately trained physical health nurses and social workers, when instructed on how to address mental health and substance-use disorders, were found to be as effective as behavioral health personnel in performing many, if not most, integrated care tasks.

If specialized psychiatric expertise for treatment of nonresponsive, complex patients or formal psychotherapy, such as cognitive behavioral therapy or interpersonal psychotherapy, was needed, then outpatient integrated care managers could refer patients to a mental health or substance-use disorder specialty clinic. This is where the lights of clinical psychologists shone brightest. Unlike days of old, however, behavioral health specialists in the medical setting and the primary and/or specialty medical physicians with whom they shared patients worked actively and closely together for the benefit of their patients. Routinely, both followed outcomes to ensure that their patients were recovering. When that did not appear to be the case, alternative approaches were discussed with each other and the patient. If necessary, off-site mental health and/or substance-use disorder providers would become involved. Correlation of the effectiveness of treatment for both medical and the behavioral conditions were routinely part of the discussion.

Early identification using ProAct and more ready availability of psychiatric consultation for patients in the inpatient setting added a dimension to care that had not been anticipated. Working in mental health teams, it was possible for nurses, social workers, and psychiatrists to support medical unit personnel in providing crisis intervention by creating mini behavior modification programs, assessing competence, suggesting and/or refining psychiatric medications, and identifying discharge resources for patients with psychiatric comorbidity.

Adequately supported, the consultation service capabilities were far superior to previous versions because they saw mainly complex, high-cost patients and were able to follow the patients through the course of the hospitalization. In the past year, they had initiated a delirium prevention service in several of the Providence hospitals that did a high volume with elective surgery and/or elderly patients.

Psychiatric services also were available in the emergency room, though they remained reactive rather than proactive. Renovation of several of the emergency suites had increased both staff and patient safety. With limited bed capacity an ongoing problem, consultation personnel had trained a number of regular emergency nursing staff to supervise psychotic and/or suicidally depressed patients when psychiatric beds were not available.

Recommendations for a centralized emergency facility were being debated citywide. Providence General was the logical location so that police and ambulances for the majority of patients would not have far to travel. The county hospital located about a mile away was a logical alternative, but they did not have as well organized or integrated inpatient capability. That, however, was changing.

HEALTH PLAN FACTOR

Mr. Romani had never questioned the cost-saving potential of coordinating treatment, especially for his members who used a disproportionate share of health care resources. As the momentum toward integration picked up, he was impressed with the detail and extent of the plan developed by the Providence health system and appreciated that mental health and substance-use disorder personnel were not only involved but also enmeshed in the medical setting.

Before committing to the project five years ago, he and Edward had done extensive analyses on claims data. Comparing the total cost of care for patients with and without behavioral health service use, including a comparison of total costs broken down into physical health, pharmacy, and mental health/substance-use disorder service between treated and untreated behavioral health users, had banished any hesitation. His board of directors had agreed to take the risk, and the risk had been rewarded.

Integration had redefined how behavioral health care was supported, and Ecumenical Care was behind the eight ball in advanced support for integrated product lines. Their internal work processes now:

- Added behavioral health procedures and treatments to health policy committee reviews.

- Cross-trained customer and provider service staff to handle both physical health and psychiatric queries.

- Combined physical and behavioral health case and disease management activities.

- Boasted mental health and substance-use disorder claims processing algorithms that simplified the adjudication process so that behavioral health and general medical were more similar than dissimilar.

- Incorporated and consolidated patient identification numbers for psychiatric claims to those for physical health.

- Importantly, processed physical and behavioral health benefits in a single budget.

The stepwise process of Ecumenical Care's leadership identified risk factors up front, addressed them, and moved forward to a new and distinguishing goal of superintegration. This included the integration of physical health and psychiatric services (level one) and the integration of care management services (level two), including case and disease management, disability management, employee assistance, workers' compensation, and health promotion.

Ecumenical Care did not just say they could do it. They did it. Edward estimated that superintegration could achieve a 5 percent net reduction in claims costs for patients with complex illness who participated in the program. With no independent behavioral health administrative infrastructure and claims adjudication process, they also had substantially reduced administrative expenses. In short, they could offer their purchasers a more competitive product.

Telstar now contracted only with Ecumenical Care and the Blues. Several other medium to large businesses either had chosen Ecumenical Care as the only health plan for their employees or had coupled it with the Blues as an option among the suite of options employees had in deciding on coverage each year. Other than the Blues, regional health plans had not moved as aggressively toward integration, such as Medical Mart. Those that did not had lost market share, experienced substantial layoffs, and were flirting with bankruptcy.

Ferdinand Behavior (FB), BVD, and other managed behavioral health organizations had slipped from 80 percent of the behavioral health market in the Denver region to 25 percent over four years and were still dropping. BVD was already in Chapter 11 bankruptcy. FB, with a national presence, was closing its doors in Colorado and looking at major restructuring nationally. A stand-alone behavioral health business could not begin to offer the benefits of an integrated program. Unfortunately for them, what was going on in Colorado had become a national trend.

Many health plans, initially taking only baby steps toward support of integrated services, were some two years behind Ecumenical Care. Attempting to get in on the action without abandoning their independently managed behavioral health operation contracts, they had unsuccessfully created work-arounds. Because the data coming out of the integrated health plan programs was too impressive to ignore, many of these timid companies now were striking outdated business procedures and prioritizing mental health and substance-use disorder treatment in the medical setting.

It was only a matter of time before the pendulum swung entirely toward integration. Collaboration between the major stakeholders of Providence Health System, Ecumenical Care, and ECI, with researchers at the University of Colorado, and eventually a grant from the National Institutes of Health had led to a telling measurement.

The differences in impairment outcomes between patients who had participated in integrated care and those who had not were impressive. There was a 5 percent cost reduction in total health care costs, but also a substantial decrease in alcohol and substance-related work absences. As well, both short- and long-term disability costs, workers' compensation claims, and family/medical leave had declined within two years of operation.

In the first six months of data collection, Vicki, Alex, and Edward had been concerned that the cost of health care actually had gone up in the patients participating in the integrated care arm of the study. But they relaxed when they realized the numbers equilibrated at 12 months and reversed at the 18-month analyses. These findings were consistent with earlier published studies, evidencing that it took six months to reverse the effects of poor clinical care (through higher cost for clinical treatment given) and another six months for patients who had recovered to get back to meaningful employment and productive activity. Thereafter, restored health was associated with reduced health care service use, decreased work absence, and increased productivity. A win for everyone.

Edward, a liaison between health plans and providers, continuously motivated product design upgrades. Through Vicki, he kept abreast of the latest innovations in clinical integration and advised Ecumenical Care on how to improve patient outcomes as a means of most efficiently using health care resources. With this background, many health plans were courting Edward to develop their own super-integration products, and the Blues, in particular, had its eye on Edward, if for no other reason than to arrest Ecumenical Care's competitive edge.

Alex, too, had countless job offers, but now director of human resources at Telstar, he was content to apply his influence from the birthplace of the initiative. Without Telstar's enormous confidence, the Integrated Physical and Behavioral Health Center of Excellence, where patients with concurrent behavioral and physical illness received top-notch treatment, could not have been realized.

The journey to integrated care had been a long and winding road, with tremendous effort extended by forward-thinking individuals who chose excellence over security in order to enhance the quality of U.S. health care. The result was a new paradigm of health care services that promised to:

- Provide excellent mental health and substance-use disorder services in general medical clinics and on general hospital units.
- Rapidly and effectively improve clinical outcomes for patients with complex and high-cost comorbid illness.
- Lower health care costs by improving clinical outcomes and reducing service use in complex patients.
- Decrease impairment and enhance greater employee productivity.

Chapter 9

INTEGRATED CARE

I want it said of me by those who knew me best, that I always plucked
a thistle and planted a flower where I thought a flower would grow.[1]
—Abraham Lincoln

Konrad Zuse, an engineering student living in Berlin, circa 1934, concluded that
the binary system was better suited for calculating numbers than the decimal system. To avoid boring mathematical calculations common to his field, he built a
binary-based calculating machine to complete his homework assignments. By
1938, and already working on the third generation of his programmable Z3, Zuse
was years ahead of George Stibitz, who developed the Complex Number Cal-
culator for Bell Laboratories in Manhattan, and Howard Aiken, designer of the
Harvard Mark I. His creative work, though isolated, was the forerunner to what is
now the billion-dollar computer industry.

Though Alex is fictional, his dedication to integrated health care represents the
selfsame pioneering spirit that infused Zuse. Alex's integrated approach promises
quality care, coordinated care, and less cost to every health system that chooses to
use it. Isolated in a large Midwest town and working for a growing business concern, he gathered a team of risk takers and dared to rattle the precarious status quo.
Gambling both reputation and livelihood, he and his colleagues refused the notion
that behavioral health was separate from the rest of health, and then, zeroing in
on one of the many-faceted components of a system spinning out of control, they
endeavored to contribute to a better health system.

Several major reports since the turn of the millennia have documented the
impact of mental illness on the lives of Americans and have tabulated present
shortcomings and opportunities for the future. Dr. David Sacher issued a call to

action with his *Mental Health: A Report of the Surgeon General* in December 1999, wherein he documents that mental health problems are prevalent and treatable but that mental health treatment is more difficult to get than physical health care and that stigma remains a barrier.[2]

Three and a half years later, under the watch of George W. Bush, the final report from the President's New Freedom Commission on Mental Health, titled *Achieving the Promise: Transforming Mental Health Care in America,* confirmed that mental health is essential to overall health.[3] The report recommended research and the use of technology to forward consumer- and family-driven improvement by fostering early intervention, access, use of evidence-based practices, and elimination of discriminatory practices in the identification and treatment of mental illness. Although the report is well written and informative, it sidesteps how the health care infrastructure would have to change in order to accomplish its recommendations. Finally, the Institute of Medicine's 2005 report titled *Improving the Quality of Health Care for Mental and Substance-Use Conditions* was published as the mental health compendium to a previous report, *Crossing the Quality Chasm: A New Health System for the 21st Century,* which focused on general medical care.[4] Expanding the suggestions of the surgeon general's and the Freedom Report, *Improving the Quality of Health Care for Mental and Substance-Use Conditions* specifically recommends that "policies and incentives increase collaboration among these (primary care, mental health, and substance-use treatment) providers to achieve evidence-based screening and care of their patients with general medical, mental, and/or substance-use health conditions."[5] The authors then go on to describe an integrated system similar to one that we have tangibly created in this book. The final and important proposal in the report states that "federal and state governments should revise laws, regulations, and administrative practices that create inappropriate barriers to the communication of information between providers of health care for mental and substance-use conditions and between those providers and providers of general care."[6]

Alex's campaign to eliminate the well-reported shortcomings of the health care system was, in many ways, equivalent to Zuse's efforts to improve computing devices. Prior to Zuse's inspiration, Charles Babbage attempted to develop an analytic engine using the decimal system (base 10), but despite an intact conceptual framework for the design and programming of a calculating machine, he was doomed to failure. Centuries later, Konrad recognized the numbering system Babbage had chosen was unsuitable to the task. Using Babbage's principle concept, he started with the supposition that the binary system (base two, i.e., using 0s and 1s) was the best way to develop a calculating machine. He succeeded. Today's computers, by relaying basic arithmetic functions, perform nearly 1 trillion floating point operations per second (FLOPS). Like Zuse, Alex with his colleagues Edward and Vicki began with a fresh but basic concept. They looked at a system of care that attempted to isolate behavioral health care from physical health care and saw that it was doomed to failure. Only by altering the system so that psychiatric illness was inherently incorporated into general medical care could real improvement in health, reduction in impairment, and lowering of health-related cost be expected.

Unlike Zuse, however, Alex lived in a world built around the thistle separating physical and behavioral illnesses. In order to realize his vision of an integrated approach to ECI employees' care, he had to recreate an infrastructure that would allow it to happen, and he knew ECI and Telstar could not pull it off alone. He had to demonstrate the value to other employers with similar interests, and because an integrated product was not currently available for purchase, he had to produce one. Few health plans possessed even a conceptual framework of what an integrated care reimbursement system for physical health and mental/substance-use disorders might look like. As well, care separation had been in existence for so long, clinical systems relied on their entrenched autonomy for profitability.

Edward and Ecumenical Care also were stymied. They could not create an integrated product in isolation. Without a purchaser base and consistent reimbursement for the clinical programs willing to set up integrated services by most if not all health plans in addition to themselves, they would have few buyers and even fewer providers to deliver integrated programs. Adverse selection would throw them into financial disarray.

Finally, Vicki only had been successful in building the inpatient medical psychiatry unit at University Hospitals because she had developed it as a medical unit. Had she done it under the administrative auspices of psychiatry, as many others had in the carved-out atmosphere, it was only a matter of time before it would be closed down. Lack of communication between physical and mental health practitioners and financial insolvency due to poor reimbursement by managed behavioral health vendors could not sustain them.

The single most glaring omission in the surgeon general's, the President's Freedom Commission, and Institute of Medicine's reports was their failure to recognize the important first step. To successfully alter treatment of concurrent general medical and psychiatric illnesses and reverse the high costs typical in complex patients, *the payment system must change.* Short of this, solutions would be locally limited or ineffective.

It all had to do with responsibility and accountability from which quality practices, provider communication, and collaboration emanate. Unless physical health practitioners see treatment of mental health and substance-use conditions as a part of their responsibility, they will continue to refer or look the other way. Likewise, behavioral health clinicians must recognize the impact that psychiatric illness has on comorbid physical conditions. Without coordination of services with primary and specialty medical physicians, both they and their physical health colleagues will have little success in reversing the suffering and pain experienced by their patients and the impact that they have on health care service use.

Fast-forwarding 15 years, let us revisit the six patients we read about in Chapter 1. Eva, Mohammed, Harry, and the others now live in a health care environment similar to that created by Alex, Edward, and Vicki. As we will see, even without anticipated major advances in treatment technologies, such as gene therapy, organ regeneration, and the like, there is great value in simple restructuring of the way that health care services are financed and supported. Proper identification and treatment of behavioral health disorders lead to improved clinical results in a more effective and efficient health care environment.

* * *

Eva sits at her computer browsing Amazon for her older son's birthday gift. Three mahogany plaques adorn the wall behind the desk: "Eva Perkins, IT Specialist of the YEAR," "Eva Perkins, Outstanding Volunteer," "Eva Perkins, President-Elect, Staff Training Operation." Her jogging sweats are tight around the waist and her ankles swell from time to time, but her complexion is rosy.

A little more than six months ago Eva's dad died, expectedly, painlessly. Shortly after the funeral, she noticed a slump in her energy. She was irritable and moody. Attributing her blue mood to losing her dad, she reconnected with Polly, the psychologist who had helped her get through her divorce five years earlier. She assured Polly that she was not feeling suicidal, "just kind of sad." Polly saw her three times to help support her through this period of grief and felt confident Eva was coming out of the slump. But to the contrary, Eva's slide had just begun.

Eva's supervisor noted a change in her work performance. This correlated with accumulating sick days tagged by the disability manager. She brought it to the attention of the occupational health nurse (OHN). Noting that Eva had consistently been a stellar employee, the OHN encouraged Eva to meet with the company's employee assistance program (EAP) counselor. Negative thoughts flitted through Eva's mind. She did not need the intrusion, but the OHN had been clear about reports of a decline in her work habits. To protect her job, she begrudging made the appointment. After hearing Eva's history of depression and diabetes and the recent death in her family, the EAP counselor, with Eva's permission, sent a summary of their meeting to both Polly and Eva's family physician.

Dr. Scott recognized immediately that it was not just an exacerbation of Eva's diabetes that had led to several visits in the past four months for poorly controlled blood sugar levels and worsening hypertension. Though Eva had been adamant that she had been adhering to her insulin therapy and eating right, the numbers said something different. At her last appointment, he had adjusted her insulin dosages and insisted that she make a log of her blood sugars. She was to schedule a follow-up in two weeks. Eva had not set up the appointment.

After assessing Eva's comprehensive records of which Polly's notes were a part, Dr. Scott restarted her on Prozac and left an intercom message for Polly whose office was in an adjacent clinic. They met for coffee in the clinic cafeteria the next morning to discuss Eva's situation and to catch up on several other common patients.

Depression is very common in diabetes. Whether this is because the brain is predisposed to low mood due to widely fluctuating glucose levels or the stress and uncertainty about having a serious and chronic health problem is unknown, but probably a combination of both, with greater risk for those who have been diagnosed with depression prior to the onset of diabetes. Regardless, Dr. Scott recognized that patients with diabetes who had even mild depression are susceptible to fatalistic attitudes, which, in turn, retard their motivation to make disciplined diabetic treatment choices.

The interaction of these two serious illnesses is well established. When diabetes is brought under control, depression is typically less prominent, if present at all. When depression is effectively treated, glucose levels are easier to control. Coordinated treatment of both is mandatory to get patients back on their feet and to avoid unnecessary complications.

For the past five years, Polly, a licensed master's-level psychologist, and Dr. Scott had discussed common patients regularly. Polly was a member of their multispecialty physician's clinic along with other psychologists, social workers, psychiatric clinical nurse specialists, and psychiatrists with a special interest in the medically ill. This allowed Polly to see Eva in the medical multi-specialty clinic for depression assessment and treatment and to be paid without the hassle of frequent and intrusive prior approvals.

Impressed by the consistently successful outcomes of cognitive therapy, Polly had long ago given up her psychoanalytic practice, which was expensive and without guarantee. She worked as a part of the team of behavioral health specialists whose task it was to support general medical practitioners in treating patients with psychiatric illness. She enjoyed being in the medical setting. It widened her circle of colleagues and gave her an appreciation for the degree to which mental health issues interacted with physical illnesses. Further, she came to realize the value of sharing her clinical notes with her physical health professional colleagues, which led to better care.

Polly discussed Eva's current circumstances and spent several weeks reestablishing the use of her prior cognitive behavioral therapy (CBT) skills. During the last depression several years earlier, Eva required hospitalization with medication in addition to cognitive behavioral therapy. At that time, poor diabetic control also was a factor. Dr. Scott already had restarted Eva on Prozac, which had been helpful in the past. Throughout the initial treatment phase, both he and Polly followed Eva closely to make sure that she took her antidepressant medication, completed her CBT homework assignments, kept current on her blood pressure and blood sugar diary, and adhered to diet and exercise recommendations. Polly's notes in the medical chart provided Dr. Scott with up-to-date progress reports. Within five weeks, he watched the Patient Health Questinnaire-9 (PHQ-9) scores come down, nicely indicating that Eva's depression was under better control. Several months later, her diabetes control indicator (HbA1c) levels also had dropped more than a percentage point.

Eva returned to the company health spa's spin class and once again started participating in her kids' school events. Now that her diabetes was under better control, Dr. Scott encouraged Eva to follow up on her eye checkup, which she did. He continued her Prozac, likening its use to her new antihypertensive medications. Even though by 12 weeks she no longer experienced symptoms of depression, the medication prevented future depressive episodes.

Polly and Dr. Scott shared updates on Eva in the clinic hall between patients and through a common clinic note system. As a courtesy, both Dr. Scott and Polly sent notes to Dr. Nicholas, the psychiatrist who had assisted with control of Eva's depression several years earlier. He had not been needed for this episode, but who knows about the future. Depression and diabetes are not a good combination.

Eva's dad's death triggered a mild depression that disrupted Eva's motivation to control her diabetes. Poorly controlled diabetes with reprimands by Dr. Scott just heightened her depression. Had this vicious circle been allowed to continue, Eva would have been at greater risk for eye, heart and blood vessel, kidney, and nerve damage, the four most common complications of diabetes. Her employer would be stuck with an unproductive employee. Medical costs would mount.

Because Polly and Dr. Scott could work together in the outpatient medicine clinic, the integrated quality health care Eva received prevented excessive and reoccurring medical bills. She was not forced to change jobs for poor performance, and her employer was not subjected to the expenses of disability insurance benefits. Dr. Scott kicked himself in retrospect because he had not tumbled to the fact that depression was involved in controlling her sugar. Why not begin doing depression screens on his diabetic patients? Hmmm!

With new behavioral skill sets to tap, Eva maintained an optimistic attitude and had her diabetes back under control. Her high-stepping energy was once again noticeable at work, and her kids were getting three squares a day. Everybody won.

* * *

Anxiety, like depression, is on the upswing in the U.S. workforce. Anxiety attacks often pose as life-threatening conditions, and if the patient does not understand the dynamics of anxiety, the survival instinct naturally will catapult him to an emergency room, often by ambulance. Emergency room visits have increased by 20 percent over the past decade, whereas the number of emergency care facilities has decreased by 15 percent nationwide, causing severe overcrowding and less than quality care.[7] Integrated health care can, once again, make a dramatic difference in the cost and care of people suffering with anxiety, whether isolated or in combination with a chronic illness, as an edited version of Alvin's story will attest.

Alvin has been mentioned throughout this book because he represents a large portion of patients in the frequent-user category. This type of person does not have the patience or often the education to wade through the linguistic diarrhea of health care benefits and disease management vendor packages. At best, he knows his insurance is the gold standard. Alvin also has situations going on that aggravate his health problems. He does not understand his illness. To admit he has health issues, and especially a mental health problem, diminishes his already fragile self-image. And he is proud. Let us see how an integrated health care framework potentially could change Alvin's trajectory.

National Waste Management's OHN, Sophia, who helps employees safely reenter the workplace after an illness or family medical leave, together with Gail, the short-term disability reviewer for WorkWell, flagged Alvin's frequent days off work for illness. After several episodes, some of which the physician's reentry notes indicated had required emergency room visits and hospital stays, Gail contacted Sophia. She was curious about what was aggravating Alvin's asthma. After a discussion with Alvin, Sophia learned that AdvancedDM, the company's disease management service, had contacted him on three occasions, but Alvin never talked with them nor had he read their asthma brochure. The brochures, like many other mailers Alvin received, went into the wastebasket.

After Alvin's last asthma episode, Sophia shared what she found out and asked Gail to see if Dr. Steven, WorkWell's medical director, could talk with Alvin's primary care physician, Dr. Julie, to see if there was any way to break the asthma attack–emergency room cycle. Gail, who was already frequently in contact with Alvin during disability claims to ensure that the correct paperwork was filled out for short-term disability (STD), obtained permission from Alvin for Dr. Steven to talk with Dr. Julie. WorkWell wanted to make sure that everything that could be done was being done to help him with his asthma.

Both Dr. Julie and Dr. Steven learned much from their conversation. Dr. Steven did not know that Alvin also suffered from anxiety and panic attacks. No question, this made his treatment complicated. Dr. Julie did not know the extent of absences experienced by Alvin nor about Waste Management's EAP and disease management capabilities. She agreed that obtaining assistance from a disease management nurse was a good idea, particularly because assessment and review of anxiety as a complicating comorbidity was included. Further, she would schedule the psychiatrist, Dr. Roy, working in her multispecialty clinic to visit with the two of them during Alvin's next clinic visit.

They arranged the consultation to take place after Alvin was in contact with Advanced DM. Hopefully, they could jump-start the process of helping Alvin get control of his asthma and anxiety. Dr. Steven suggested that Alvin take several weeks of STD to complete the initial assessment and education by Advanced DM and to get on a maintenance program for his illnesses. This would impress on Alvin the importance Waste Management placed on his health.

Dr. Julie noted that last year she had tried to get him to go see someone at the local behavioral health clinic. He had gone once and said that he would never go again. Since then, Dr. Roy had come on board. Dr. Roy and Dr. Julie recommended a nurse care manager in the clinic to answer patient questions and to make sure that other factors did not interfere with Alvin's following the treatments suggested.

Dr. Julie and Dr. Roy saw Alvin in clinic 10 days later. By this time, Gail had been in contact with Alvin about Dr. Steven's and Dr. Julie's conversation. She asked Alvin if she could get a disease manager from AdvancedDM on the phone. This was much less threatening than calling himself or taking a call from someone he did not know. After a small amount of chitchat, it was possible for Gail to sign off and Alvin to continue with Mollie at AdvancedDM.

Mollie assessed Alvin for complications of asthma, including anxiety and depression. She then went through the asthma education materials, his symptoms, his treatments, and the support he received from his doctors during several 30-minute phone calls. She said that she would continue to call periodically until things were stable. Alvin liked Mollie. Unlike Dr. Julie, she was interested in him, not just his illness, and took the time to talk to him about what was really bothering him. With Mollie's help, he might be able to curb attacks and defuse Dr. Julie's frustration.

Mollie sent a note to Dr. Julie describing her first interaction with Alvin. According to Mollie, if the anxiety was presented as a common complication of asthma, seeing Dr. Roy should not be a problem. The examination and meeting with Dr. Roy went well. Alvin was now ready to take his asthma medications even when his breathing was okay. Further, Dr. Roy had explained to Alvin's satisfaction how anxiety could make asthma worse and that treatment with a medication was helpful in decreasing problems with it. Alvin was relieved to know that Dr. Julie also could manage the anxiety treatment in her clinic with the help of Dr. Roy. Alvin did not need to go to the "crazy" clinic, as his coworkers had described it.

To breathe more easily every day, an asthma sufferer must learn to work with the disease instead of fighting it. As part of Alvin's health care benefit package, he was able to access Mollie, the disease manager, who could provide the education and support needed to do so. She helped him understand the importance of controlling both the asthma and the anxiety. Drs. Julie and Roy cemented the deal through coordination of medical and psychiatric treatment. Alvin was back to work within three weeks. With Mollie's help, he took his medication regularly, was tested for potential workplace allergies, attended to early breathing symptoms, and showed up for his slightly more frequent follow-up appointments as control was established.

During the next six months, Alvin had a perfect attendance record. His coworkers no longer dreaded being on his duty assignment. In fact, they now saw Alvin as a regular guy, not the laggard they previously thought he was.

With a psychiatrist available in the medicine clinic to help Dr. Julie address Alvin's anxiety and self-esteem issues as they cropped up, control was much improved—a one-stop shop where asthma and anxiety were treated on par. No separate clinic to draw attention to Alvin's problems, no separate billing to confuse him. An investment in integrated care for Alvin yielded a healthy productive employee for National Waste Management and one less body in an overcrowded emergency room.

To have a few drinks to calm anxiety or momentarily numb depression is routine. So is having a few drinks to celebrate or grieve, to relax or turn on. Drinking is commonplace in the social fabric of U.S. life. It is also a far-reaching problem, growing more so by the tick of the clock. Alcoholism and substance-use disorders cut across the strata of ethnicity, education, and income and are no less at home in corporate offices as in transient shopping-cart communities. According to the National Clearinghouse of Alcohol and Drug Information, the loss to companies in the United States due to alcohol and drug-related use disorders totals more than $100 billion a year. Yet in a recent study examining the quality of health care for 25 common conditions, care for patients with alcohol dependence ranked last.[8]

These staggering costs do not reflect the pain and suffering aspects that can not be measured in economic terms. Take, for example, Harry from Chapter 1. The availability of appropriate intervention for Harry's alcoholism could have diverted the burden of a liver transplant and the threat to his life. In fact, Harry under the right care at the right time could have avoided a diseased liver altogether.

Harry was popping beer tabs with his buddies when he was the popular running back on his high school football team. A buckskin flask road over his shoulder on hunting trips, and a well-stocked cooler on a camping trip was as important as dry kindling. He was the life of the party, a generous and witty drunk. He married his high school sweetheart, secured a great job at Capitol Industries, bought a beautiful home, and filled it with children. Then one day, Harry's gut began to gnaw.

Eventually, Dr. Ken, Harry's general practitioner (GP), diagnosed an ulcer. As a part of the routine examination, he screened Harry about his drinking habits using the CAGE alcohol dependence screening instrument, which indicated signs of alcohol dependence (alcoholism). Dr. Ken prided himself on keeping up with the literature. He had been impressed with the results of studies on screening and brief intervention (SBI) for early alcoholism, which was designed to be provided by GPs for people just like Harry (Table 2.4). Using this simple technique, alcohol use is reduced and hospitalizations and emergency department visits occur less frequently than in those who do not receive it.

The technique is especially useful in patients who experience alcohol-related medical problems, such as Harry (in his early stages), but who do not necessarily need to be referred to an addiction treatment specialist and may not need to stop drinking completely. Interestingly, it had been found to be effective up to four years after the two-session counseling.[9] He gave Harry the alcohol-use pamphlets and spent 15 minutes discussing how this related to Harry. A follow-up appointment three weeks later was scheduled, and his nurse manager was alerted to the need for reinforcement calls. Even if Harry did not curtail his drinking, the fact that Dr. Ken had taken these steps meant that Harry was more likely to enter a formal alcohol treatment program in the future, if needed.

Five years earlier, Capitol Industries deleted the option to exclude alcohol and substance-use disorder assessment and treatment from their health plan benefit package. Although Harry did not need it at the time he took out the policy, coverage was available just as it was for cancer or heart disease. Based on solid studies, such as one on the integration of medical and substance-use disorder treatment (Table 5.3), Capitol Industries had been convinced by their health plan that it actually cost more in total health care cost if they excluded it.

The counseling of Dr. Ken and his staff brought Harry's brush with the medical complications of too much alcohol home to him. Harry never really had thought of it the way they presented it. He was not an alcoholic but knew that he was at risk because his father, uncle, and cousin all suffered the consequences of too much drinking. Although he did not completely stop his alcohol intake, he watched it closer and found that it did not impair his ability to have fun. Further, his health and his sex life had improved because he was not on the sauce so much.

Dr. Ken's progressive treatment had prevented Harry from life-threatening liver failure, and in turn, Harry's adherence to Dr. Ken's recommendations had protected his kids' college fund. By not excluding alcohol and substance-abuse treatment from their benefit package, Capitol Industries had saved several hundred thousand dollars for a liver transplantation. As a result, they had lower premiums and could cover employees with higher-risk conditions who were less responsive to preventive measures. An added bonus was a more productive workforce.

* * *

Eva, Alvin, and Harry are employees, and because employers are the major purchasers of health care services, how employees spend health care dollars are benchmarks in assessing the health and well-being of the health care system. To no degree, however, are dollars the sole measure.

Also falling into the frequent-user category are nonemployees. Some are dependents; some are in public programs. One of the many unintended consequences of managed care has been the extreme reduction in the availability of behavioral health care professionals, especially in the field of child psychiatry. With the explosion of childhood depression, attention-deficit/hyperactivity disorder (ADHD), and autistic disorders, the subsequent elevated numbers of children on prescription drugs recently have put the spotlight on treatment efficacy and/or accurate diagnoses with big questions to answer. Are we blindly drugging our children? If some children and adolescents truly would benefit from medication, are we giving them to the right kids for the right reasons?

When he was a little boy, Mohammed cuddled and clung. His dad called him "mommy's boy." After the twins were born, he became weepy and withdrawn. On Mohammed's first day of kindergarten, Mrs. Zar had to pry him out of the car. He protested, "Why was I ever born?" By third grade, he was interrupting the teacher, squabbling with his classmates, and refusing to obey the rules. Though his national test scores were high, his grades were dismal. At home, from one minute to the next, Mohammed's moods swung from despair to glee. He slept no more than four to six hours a night yet was a bolt of energy the next day.

By the time Mohammed was 11 years old, Mrs. Zar knew her son was different from the other kids, and though her husband wrote off the escalating bad behavior as so-called growing pains, she overrode her husband's objections and called their pediatrician. Gleaned from information she had read off the Internet and from magazine articles, she felt sure Mohammed had some sort of mental imbalance.

Mania in children often looks like hyperactivity and excitability, and one of the biggest challenges to pediatricians is to differentiate children with bipolar illness from those with ADHD. Dr. John, with limited exposure to behavioral, as opposed to physical, development as part of his medical school and residency training, was familiar with bipolar disease but had few patients whom he had diagnosed and treated.

He was, however, very familiar with ADHD and had treated many ADHD patients with methylphenidate (Ritalin) and other stimulant medications. Because Mohammed's symptoms were a bit different than a usual ADHD condition, and recognizing that any delay in appropriate treatment would be costly, he decided to talk with Dr. Jerry, the new child psychiatrist who had moved in down the hall.

Dr. Jerry had arrived in the multispecialty pediatric clinic about six months earlier. Because billing and coding rules had changed several years earlier, he could work in the pediatric clinic without hassle. Further, he was able to hire a pediatric clinical nurse specialist with an interest in psychiatry while another was being oriented. This had substantially extended the number of patients he was able to assist and pleased his pediatric colleagues. They had been starving for support.

Though his schedule was no less hectic than it had been at the stand-alone Metropolitan Child and Adolescent Psychiatry offices, he now could call on the pediatricians for advice and assistance with some of his more complicated patients. Perhaps more importantly, they could call on him. He and his team of psychologists, nurses, and social workers were able to take care of things that the pediatricians were not. The pediatricians for their part participated in treatment plans once they had been well developed and under way. It was a good arrangement, one that he thought he could sell to the other child psychiatrists he was recruiting.

Within five minutes, Dr. Jerry knew that Mohammed was a complicated case. Dr. John shared the story, noting the mood swings, the history of depression in both Mr. and Mrs. Zar's family, and the symptom onset and progression. He told Dr. John to call his nurse clinician to do an accelerated evaluation, available only to the pediatricians in the clinic, later that day. The evaluation was performed by one of the intake psychologist team members. Dr. Jerry reviewed the findings with the psychologist and set the wheels in motion for a complete assessment and, ultimately, treatment.

In the meantime, Mr. and Mrs. Zar were given suggestions on how to manage Mohammed while the work-up was in progress. Because Mohammed was not actively suicidal, there was time to complete the evaluation. Within several weeks, based on symptoms described and confirmed by family and the school nurse, Mohammed was diagnosed with bipolar illness. A treatment program was developed that included a combination of supportive therapy for Mohammed, training in management techniques for Mr. and Mrs. Zar, development of limit-setting procedures and of support for Mohammed's teachers, and a mood stabilizer.

Though he still had problems, Mohammed gradually came under better control. When Mohammed's behavior and medication management were stabilized, he was transferred to Dr. John, who would have ready access to Dr. Jerry if problems arose. Dr. Jerry would continue to see Mohammed intermittently, as would other members of the mental health team, and Dr. John would provide routine follow-up.

Margie's story in Chapter 1 explores the curious population of patients with unexplained somatic complaints (USCs). Margie has lots of symptoms that, naturally, her doctors take seriously. She gets evaluated, referred, and treated aggressively and often. Cost estimates place somatization disorder in the same rank as end-stage liver disease and ovarian cancer.

In a given year, Americans with frequent somatic symptoms make an estimated 150 million unnecessary doctor visits and 17 million unnecessary emergency room visits. They account for 2 million unnecessary hospital admissions. Research on these patients suggests that their annual health care costs for unnecessary encounters range somewhere between $10 billion and $20 billion.[10] Each of these encounters puts patients at risk because tests, medications, and other treatment can cause adverse reactions and complications.

Of course, all unnecessary medical treatments can not be pinned on patients like Margie, but patients like her rack up a troubling sum of wasted health care resources. In Margie's case, her husband's company health plan picks up the tab after deduction maximums are reached. Her high service use, however, ultimately shifts to the public by way of higher premiums and taxes. In Chapter 1, Margie received no psychiatric intervention because in the nonintegrated system there was little opportunity or interest in rocking the medical boat. Testing and treatment is, after all, a cash cow. But provider profit motivation was not the only blockade. Patients do not usually respond well to suggestions that their symptoms may not be related to physical illness, and Margie was no exception.

Margie doted on her husband and fussed over her toddler. She chatted freely in grocery store checkout lanes about the latest wrinkle creams and the price of tomatoes. She volunteered her time to the Altar Society and walked the neighborhood for the March of Dimes. She knew who was having a baby and who was having an affair. She also knew every doctor and nurse who lived and breathed in her hometown of El Dorado as well as in the bordering metropolis, Wichita. In fact, she knew them in Kansas City and St. Louis and Boston.

Dr. Keith, the medical director at Coastal Care, the health plan that handled Margie's health benefits, had approved countless exploratory surgeries, X-rays, scopings, angiograms, and biopsies on her behalf in years past. In the last 20 years, she had been to 29 different primary care physicians, 14 stomach specialists, 8 heart specialists, 6 gynecologists, a urologist, 11 skin specialists, and numerous health care support specialists, such as physical therapists, optometrists, chiropractors, naturopaths, and acupuncturists. Emergency room visits and hospitalization had been routine. After the birth of her daughter, Dr. Keith noticed a spike in medical service use, including a couple of trips to an expensive medical center on the East Coast.

Her turnaround began when she was admitted to Hutchison Hospital nearly 12 years ago while visiting relatives. Even with her stomach pain off the charts, a physical examination, blood tests, and abdominal X-rays had revealed nothing other than a diffusely tender stomach. Informed by her husband about Margie's extensive health problems and the multiple scopings that had never uncovered abnormalities, her doctors decided an endoscopic retrograde cholangiopancreatography (ERCP—a fancy bile duct test) was potentially necessary. Because the Hutchinson doctors were out of Margie's physician network, prior approval was necessary for most expensive procedures, and Dr. Keith was called.

Having learned much about somatization disorder during the introduction of integrated care, Dr. Keith confirmed the absence of objective medical findings and suggested a conservative approach because he knew that her symptoms typically improved within 24 hours, though they never went away completely. He indicated that as soon as she was stable, her doctors should send her, by ambulance if necessary, to Baptist Hospital in Wichita, where they had opened an integrated inpatient unit in the last six months. Unless they did so, in the absence of objective abnormalities on physical examination and medical testing, he could not approve payment for the admission or any procedures they may choose to perform.

Margie and her husband called Dr. Keith immediately when they heard of the requirement for transfer. Standing firm on his recommendation, Dr. Keith said that they certainly could stay at the hospital in Hutchison if they wished and her doctors there could proceed with any test they considered necessary, but without approved payment. He made it clear that with Margie's history of medical problems, he considered it important for her to be treated in the complex care unit at the Baptist Hospital in Wichita, which had a special interest in patients with problems such as Margie's. He assured them that there was access to the full range of health services in the unit.

To the relief of the doctors, an angry and confused Margie was delivered by ambulance to the integrated inpatient unit in Wichita, where she was admitted, evaluated by an internal medicine specialist and a psychiatrist, treated for symptoms using conservative measures, and observed. Perhaps the most important part of Margie's admission was the thorough review of the extensive faxed records that Margie had accumulated and discussions with the doctors who had taken care of her, family physicians, internists, surgeons, and many other medical specialists.

Margie had several identifiable objective medical conditions, such as an accessory spleen, high blood fats, periodic urinary tract infections, and a history of repeated infections with streptococcal pharyngitis. She also had more than 45 separate symptoms for which she had received an evaluation, test, referral, or medication for which no illness was uncovered. In addition to the few objective medical illnesses, Margie's records were replete with medication intolerances and testing complications. In many ways, Margie was her own worst enemy. She had a tendency to overreact to symptoms, seek medical attention, and then suffer complications from the tests and treatments that the doctors gave.

Initially, during admission to the integrated treatment unit, Margie complained about all the rules and bristled that the unit door needed to be locked because there were confused patients admitted there. By the time of discharge, however, she was pleased with the attention she had been given by the doctors and nurses. Some of the best treatment she had every gotten, she said, "People seemed to listen here."

During the course of hospitalization, Margie was taken off of 5 medications and told to throw away an additional 15 in her medicine cabinet that she took when she needed them—her just-in-case meds. She would be encouraged to cut down on several others over the next several months by the doctors who followed her progress.

While in the hospital, as predicted by Dr. Keith, Margie's symptoms lessened with nonspecific treatment (nonsteroidal anti-inflammatory agents, antacids, and walking). From day one, she was encouraged to become involved in the unit's communal activities. She appreciated the thoroughness with which her records were reviewed. Her inclusive physical examination and the doctors' willingness to listen to descriptions of her symptoms gave her confidence in her medical team. In the course of her treatment, she learned that she did not have a serious illness and that eating a well-balanced, nonrestricted diet and exercise would help, not hinder, her health. She learned that the many medications she was taking could be contributing to her symptoms, and that very possibly her stomach problems would continue to get better and eventually go away if she chose her medications prudently.

Along with this simple advice came the second salvo: Stick with one doctor and follow her or his advice even though testing and medication may not be included in the medical recommendations. If she did not have a doctor with whom she felt comfortable, the doctors on the unit could arrange for her to be seen in the new complex-patient outpatient program at their multispecialty medical clinic. She opted for the latter because the doctors in El Dorado seemed to have little interest in her any longer, and Wichita was only a 30-minute drive.

Years ago, Margie's medical bill tallied as much as $70,000 annually. Within an integrated system, Margie's treatment was not only more effective but also far less expensive. Receiving the right care, her medical claims dropped dramatically during the first year in the integrated care clinic. Over the intervening years, they remained only a third more than other patients her age with similar health conditions but substantially lower than before her fateful admission to the medical psychiatry unit. Her pill bottles disappeared from her medicine cabinets, and with less of her energy focused on health issues, Margie flourished. She still took more time during clinic visits and needed to be seen every two to four weeks, but with this type of attention, health crises were averted. Simply, Margie now had more time for interests and family because less time was devoted to health issues.

* * *

Margie's care described how a coordinated general medical and psychiatric inpatient unit can reduce the need for a person plagued with illness concerns to seek treatment. Mrs. Abraham's situation will illustrate the advantage brought to patients with active and concurrent physical (ulcer) and mental health (delirium) symptoms, which retard the ability of quality physicians and nursing personnel to provide efficient outcome-changing care. In fact, our Mrs. Abraham from Chapter 1 was lucky that she did not suffer further injury or even death while receiving treatment in the traditional setting in which doctors are trained to focus on illnesses in their own domain, whether medical or psychiatric, and are unable to coordinate them because of the separation of intervention expectations.

Usually a nice little lady, friendly to all, Mrs. Abraham had suddenly turned nasty. A longtime resident of The Commons, she had become progressively confused, pulling stunts uncharacteristic of her. Over the last couple of weeks, she rarely showed up for meals, and when she did, she got belligerent with residents if they tried to sit at her table. She spit at facility staff with slight, and often no, provocation. Usually fastidious in both hygiene and fashion, she refused to bathe herself, comb her hair, or change her clothes. The morning she barricaded her apartment door for fear of being molested, the nursing staff knew it was time to take action.

At the request of Mrs. Abraham's children who lived out of state, the assisted-living facility nurse ordered an ambulance to take their mother to Mercy Hospital, where a complex-patient unit was available. Following the unit's inception seven years earlier, many residents from The Commons had used its services, where they had received excellent care.

Jennifer, the triage nurse in the emergency room, knew that Mrs. Abraham would require immediate attention and close observation. From the behavior profile the facility nurse had described over the phone, Jennifer anticipated that Mrs. Abraham was destined for the psychiatry unit, where control of her combative and abusive behavior would be possible. She, however, had a lingering concern because the stress of even a minor medical illness in an elderly person with memory difficulties like Mrs. Abraham could be a trigger for the onset of delirium, a condition suggested by the nursing home report. A thorough physical assessment would be critical.

Despite Mrs. Abraham's hostile demeanor and shrill objections, informed consent obtained from family members by The Commons staff nurse allowed an examination to be completed within 10 minutes of reaching the emergency room. Blood was drawn, a urine sample obtained, and symptoms consistent with delirium documented.[11] It took nearly two hours, with Mrs. Abraham in soft restraints and under constant observation, for the results of the lab tests to show that Mrs. Abraham was anemic, but not dangerously so. Dark brown stool found in the patient's undergarments had also been positive for trace blood. Although stool testing would need repeating, the first order of business was to stabilize Mrs. Abraham's behavior.

Years earlier, Mercy Hospital had used the intensive care unit to control patients like Mrs. Abraham, and long stays were the standard. Now all that had changed. She was whisked from the emergency room to the complex care unit, where nurses and other unit staff treated delirious patients regularly. She was placed near the nursing station in a quiet single room with a calendar, clock, and soft music. The room also was equipped with a video camera, like others of its kind on the unit, so that delirious, suicidal, or unpredictable patients needing close monitoring could be observed by one member of the nursing staff from central monitors in the nursing station. All nurses were trained in behavior-control techniques, rendering long-term restraints unusual.

It was important that Mrs. Abraham's behavior be controlled quickly so that the cause of her anemia could be assessed while protecting her from her own agitation and confusion. The unit was under the supervision of both an internist and a psychiatrist. The two worked as a team to ensure quick, safe, and legal care. One nurse was assigned to help soothe Mrs. Abraham's agitation through both personal support and, under the guidance of the physician team, the aggressive use of intramuscular and intravenous medication known to work for delirium.

Within three hours, Mrs. Abraham was asleep but able to be roused. During this much-needed rest, something she had not had for nearly five days, it was possible to repeat her blood count and the stool test for blood (guaiac). Her anemia was mild, so a transfusion was unnecessary, but stool continued to demonstrate the presence of blood. She needed to have a tube snaked through her mouth into her stomach (gastroscopy), which allowed the doctors to look at her stomach lining in the event that a slow-bleeding ulcer was causing her problem. Permission was obtained through a monitored phone call to Mrs. Abraham's oldest son, her medical power of attorney. Support for the procedure was confirmed by her daughter, who had just flown in from the coast.

When Mrs. Abraham awoke, much of her confusion had dissipated. She was not sure how she had gotten to the hospital but was pleased to see her daughter. The tranquilizing medications had done their job. As a result, it had long ago been possible to discontinue the protective soft restraints. She was told of the need for the scoping procedure. With the help of the daughter, tacit permission from her also was obtained.

While Mrs. Abraham was under sedation, the uncomplicated procedure revealed a small bleeding ulcer. Considering surgery unnecessary, her medical team started antacids and omeprazole, a stomach acid inhibitor. A call to the nursing home revealed that Mrs. Abraham's arthritis had kicked up several months ago. The nurses noted that she had been taking more pain medications for this. Unfortunately, these medications had the common side effect of stomach irritation and ulcers. Medications for arthritis without this side effect were started along with ulcer treatment and continued medication to control confusion. Mrs. Abraham was discharged four days after admission. Follow-up visits with the internist and psychiatrist were scheduled because it was likely that both the ulcer and confusion medication could be tapered and discontinued as her ulcer healed and confusion dissipated.

The Common's nursing staff was pleased to see her returned home so quickly and back to her pleasant self. The picture of Mrs. Abraham's illness and recovery was one they had seen many times before. Something as simple as a small stomach ulcer could tip fragile, mildly demented residents into a confused state that was in many ways more debilitating and dangerous than the medical illness that caused it. They appreciated that the addition of the complex care unit at Mercy Hospital now turned around those experiencing these problems quickly and effectively. Behavior control was a standard part of physical health care on the unit, thus patients who used to take weeks to recover, often with attendant complications, were now released almost in the same amount of time as those in whom psychiatric complications were not present. Further, follow-up was excellent. Mrs. Abraham probably would not even remember going to the hospital.

* * *

Eva, Harry, Mrs. Abraham, and the others that you met in Chapter 1 suffered with a combination of physical and psychiatric illness and were treated in a traditional care environment. Their stories are commonplace in our current system and the economic burden of their care heavy. In this chapter, their treatment took place within an integrated health care system to illustrate the extraordinary difference in both effectiveness and quality of care received when coordination of physical health and mental health/substance-use disorder exists.

In this book I have attempted to draw attention to the inadequacies of our fractured health system and to offer solutions that would allow some of the most costly and debilitated patients to avoid and/or recover from many of the ravages of combined illness. Early, effective, and efficient treatment in an integrated setting not only affords improved personal health but also strengthens interaction with family and friends, advances work productivity, and invigorates success at life interests.

It has not been my intent to suggest that by connecting physical health and mental health/substance-use disorder treatment that other limitations within the U.S. and other health systems will resolve. Integration of general medical and psychiatric intervention is just one component of the complex health care reform effort. Tackled in isolation, it would not be sufficient to turn the tide; however, discussion and policy on integration should be an integral part of every health reform debate.

Without effectively dealing with mental health and substance-use disorders as they influence the onset, progression, and treatment of protean physical health problems, and vice versa, ample evidence now demonstrates that complex patients will continue to remain physically and emotionally ill. For a long time to come, they will use high levels of health care resources and routinely drain disability and social service coffers unless steps are taken to address their plights.

Healing Body AND Mind: A Critical Issue for Health Care Reform opened with Nellie Bly's story. An investigative reporter in the late 1800s, Bly uncovered the ubiquitous abuses in mental health treatment. Since then, no doubt, we have taken giant steps forward in psychiatric care with the introduction of humane management in hospitals and outpatient settings and of treatments, such as medication, electroconvulsive therapy, and selective psychotherapies. In fact, many of today's interventions for psychiatric illness are as effective and readily available as are interventions for ulcers, high cholesterol, asthma, and diabetes.

These advances, however, have been eclipsed by poor decisions made on behalf of the mentally ill. Perhaps one of the more egregious back steps was deinstitutionalization. Lacking long-range vision, no outpatient infrastructure was created to support the vulnerable sufferers of psychiatric disorders, which has, once again, led to criminalization of the mentally ill.

In 2006, Pete Earley, also an investigative reporter, wrote an account reflecting his bipolar son's experience using the Miami Dade County Jail as the backdrop—a story that eerily mirrors Nellie Bly's.[12] In his book *Crazy: A Father's Search through America's Mental Health Madness,* Earley exposes how patients with behavioral disorders find themselves incarcerated rather than hospitalized. Housed with the general prison population, they are abused by both jail attendants and criminal detainees and receive poor, if any, treatment.

In short, other than the pay-per-view invitation extended by Bedlam administrators to London's citizenry a hundred years ago, nothing really has changed. In a supposedly modern civilized nation, a staggering number of patients with psychiatric disorders have been returned to cells and shackled as criminals. With dramatic improvements in our ability to help patients with mental health and substance-use disorders, it is difficult for me, and hopefully for the citizens of this country, to justify such injustice.

With the advent of effective treatment for many mental health and substance-use disorders, whether associated with physical illness or not, it is time to revamp the health system and destroy the barriers that perpetuate isolated treatment of body *and* mind. The body and mind cannot be separated, and only through coordination of behavioral and physical health care can good health be realized.

NOTES

CHAPTER 1

1. J.F. Kennedy, American University Commencement Address, Washington, DC, 1963, paragraph 9.

2. B. Kroeger, *Nellie Bly: Daredevil, Reporter, Feminist* (New York: Random House, 1995).

3. M. Cuneo, *American Exorcism: Expelling Demons in the Land of Plenty* (New York: Doubleday, 2001).

4. G. Amorth, *An Exorcist Tells His Story* (Fort Collins, CO: Ignatius Press, 1999).

5. R.G. Kathol, D. McAlpine, Y. Kishi, R. Spies, W. Meller, T. Bernhardt, S. Eisenberg, K. Folkert, & W. Gold. "General Medical and Pharmacy Claims Expenditures in Users of Behavioral Health Services," *Journal of General Internal Medicine* 20, no. 2 (2005): 160–67.

CHAPTER 2

1. J. Bronowski, *The Ascent of Man* (Boston: Little Brown, 1974).

2. A. Scull, C. MacKenzie, and N. Hervey, *Masters of Bedlam* (Princeton, NJ: Princeton University Press, 1996).

3. D.B. Weiner, "'Le geste de Pinel': The History of a Psychiatric Myth," in *Discovering the History of Psychiatry,* ed. M.S. Micale and R. Porter (New York: Oxford University Press, 1994), 232–47.

4. J. Suttcliffe and N. Duin, *A History of Medicine: From Prehistory to the Year 2020* (New York: Barnes and Noble Books, 1992).

5. P.C.A. Louis, *Researches on the Effects of Bloodletting in Some Inflammatory Diseases* (Boston: Hilliary, Gray, 1836).

6. J.B. Moseley, K. O'Malley, N.J. Petersen, T.J. Menke, B.A. Brody, D.H. Kuykendall, J.C. Hollingsworth, C.M. Ashton, and N.P. Wray, "A Controlled Trial of Arthroscopic

Surgery for Osteoarthritis of the Knee," *New England Journal of Medicine* 347, no. 2 (2002): 81–88.

7. American Psychiatric Association, *Diagnostic and Statistical Manual of Mental Disorders (DSM-IV-TR),* 4th ed., text rev. (Washington, DC: American Psychiatric Press, 2000).

8. H. Lavretsky and L. H. Nguyen, "Innovations: Geriatric Psychiatry: Diagnosis and Treatment of Neuropsychiatric Symptoms in Alzheimer's Disease," *Psychiatric Services* 57, no. 5 (2006): 617–19.

9. J. Caplehorn and J. J. Deeks, "A Critical Appraisal of the Australian Comparative Trial of Methadone and Buprenorphine Maintenance," *Drug and Alcohol Review* 25, no. 2 (2006): 157–60.

10. R. F. Anton, S. S. O'Malley, D. A. Ciraulo, R. A. Cisler, D. Couper, D. M. Donovan, D. R. Gastfriend, J. D. Hosking, B. A. Johnson, J. S. LoCastro et al., "Combined Pharmacotherapies and Behavioral Interventions for Alcohol Dependence: The COMBINE Study: A Randomized Controlled Trial," *Journal of the American Medical Association* 295, no. 17 (2006): 2003–17.

11. C. Weisner, J. Mertens, S. Parthasarathy, C. Moore, and Y. Lu, "Integrating Primary Medical Care with Addiction Treatment: A Randomized Controlled Trial," *Journal of the American Medical Association* 286, no. 14 (2001): 1715–23.

CHAPTER 3

1. R. McCloskey, U.S. State Department Noon Briefing, March 31, 1984.

2. M. Stobbe, "U.S. Life Expectancy Hits All-Time High," *Breitbart.com/Associated Press* (accessed December 16, 2006). http://www.breitbart.com/news/2005/12/08/D8ECE2TGD.html

3. S. Heffler, S. Smith, S. Keehan, C. Borger, M. K. Clemens, and C. Truffer, "U.S. Health Spending Projections for 2004–2014," *Health Affairs (Project Hope)* Web exclusives (2005, Suppl.): W5-74–W75-85.

4. R. Kathol and D. Clarke, "Rethinking the Place of the Psyche in Health: Toward the Integration of Healthcare Systems," *Australian and New Zealand Journal of Psychiatry* 39 (2005): 826–35.

5. D. U. Himmelstein, E. Warren, D. Thorne, and S. Woolhandler, "Illness and Injury as Contributors to Bankruptcy," *Health Affairs (Project Hope)* Web exclusives (2005, Suppl.): W5-63–W65-73.

6. C. Hoffman, A. Carbaugh, H. Y. Moore, and A. Cook, *Kaiser Commission on Medicaid and the Uninsured—Health Insurance Coverage in America: 2004 Data Update* (Washington, DC: Kaiser Family Foundation Publication, 2005).

7. K. Kiser, "Doctoring the Old-Fashioned Way," *Minnesota Medicine* 89 (January 2006; accessed December 16, 2006). http://www.mmaonline.net/Publications/MNMed2006/January/pulse%201.html

8. R. Goetzel, R. Ozminkowski, V. Villagra, and J. Duffy, "Return on Investment in Disease Management: A Review," *Health Care Financing Review* 26, no. 4 (Summer 2005): 1–19.

9. Hay Group, "Health Care Plan Design and Cost Trends: 1988 through 1998," *Haygroup* (April 1999), (accessed December 16, 2006) http://www.naphs.org/News/hay99/hay99.html

10. Kaiser Family Foundation, "Employer Health Benefits," *Kaiser Family Foundation and Health Research and Educational Trust,* 2005, http://www.kff.org/insurance (accessed December 16, 2006).

11. R. Kathol, "Pithiatism: Lost but Not Forgotten," *Psychiatric Medicine* 6 (1988): 17–21.

12. A. Ring, C.F. Dowrick, G.M. Humphris, J. Davies, and P. Salmon, "The Somatising Effect of Clinical Consultation: What Patients and Doctors Say and Do Not Say When Patients Present Medically Unexplained Physical Symptoms," *Social Science Medicine* 61, no. 7 (2005): 1505–15.

13. B.G. Druss, R.A. Rosenheck, and W.H. Sledge, "Health and Disability Costs of Depressive Illness in a Major U.S. Corporation," *American Journal of Psychiatry* 157, no. 8 (August 2000): 1274–78.

14. D.R. Jones, C. Macias, P.J. Barreira, W.H. Fisher, W.A. Hargreaves, and C.M. Harding, "Prevalence, Severity, and Co-occurrence of Chronic Physical Health Problems of Persons with Serious Mental Illness," *Psychiatric Services* 55, no. 11 (2004): 1250–57.

CHAPTER 4

1. Hippocrates, *Epidemics,* Book 1, Section XI (400 B.C.E.).

2. Kaiser Family Foundation, "Employer Health Benefits," *Kaiser Family Foundation and Health Research and Educational Trust,* http://www.kff.org/insurance (accessed April 2, 2006).

3. C. Smith, C. Cowan, A. Sensenig, and A. Catlin, "Health Spending Growth Slows in 2003," *Health Affairs* 24, no. 1 (2006): 185–94.

4. C. DeNavas-Walt, B. Proctor, and C. Lee, "Income, Poverty, and Health Insurance Coverage in the United States: 2004," *U.S. Census Bureau,* http://www.nchc.org/facts/coverage.shtml (accessed April 2, 2006).

5. M.E. Porter and E.O. Teisberg, "Redefining Competition in Health Care," *Harvard Business Review* 82, no. 6 (2004): 65–76.

6. Committee on Quality of Health Care In America. *Crossing the Quality Chasm: A New Health System for the 21st Century (Chasm Report).* Washington, DC: National Academy Press, 2001.

7. D. Ackman, "Health Care Costs More, but People Buy More," *Forbes* (2005) www.forbes.com/2005/06/21/healthcare-insurance-medicine-cx_da_0621topnews_print.html

8. P.B. Ginsburg, "Competition in Health Care: Its Evolution over the Past Decade," *Health Affairs (Project Hope)* 24, no. 6 (2005): 1512–22.

9. W. Moyer, "Baby Boomers Turn 60," *Press and Sun-Bulletin* (January 1, 2006). www.pressconnects.com/apps/pbcs.dll/article?AID=/20060101/NEWS01/601010321/006 (accessed January 17, 2006).

10. D. Thomas, "Do Not Go Gentle into That Goodnight" (1952).

11. The name *Blues* is used—here and throughout the text—as a pseudonym for several large medical managed care organizations that insure many patients in today's health care markets. Since this is a fictionalized case, no actual company name has been specified nor is any such specification intended.

12. Lyric Wallwork Winik. "Intelligence Report: Are Your Pills Making You Sick?" *Parade Magazine* (March 12, 2006).

CHAPTER 5

1. R.Z. Goetzel, S.R. Long, R.J. Ozminkowski, K. Hawkins, S. Wang, and W. Lynch, "Health, Absence, Disability, and Presenteeism Cost Estimates of Certain Physical and Mental Health Conditions Affecting U.S. Employers," *Journal of Occupational and Environmental Medicine* 46, no. 4 (2004): 398–412.

2. J. Warner, "Employers/Employees See Depression Differently," *WebMD Medical News,* (accessed March 22, 2004). www.webmd.com/content/article/84/98087.htm?printing=true

3. K. Tyler, "Mind Matters: Reducing Mental Health Care Coverage Today May Cost You More Tomorrow," *HR Magazine* 48, no. 8 (August, 2003). http://www.shrm.org/hrmagazine/articles/0803/0803tyler_benefits.asp

4. R. C. Kessler, O. Demler, R. G. Frank, M. Olfson, H. A. Pincus, E. E. Walters, P. Wang, K. B. Wells, and A. M. Zaslavsky , "Prevalence and Treatment of Mental Disorders, 1990 to 2003," *New England Journal of Medicine* 352, no. 24 (2005): 2515–23; K. Demyttenaere, R. Bruffaerts, J. Posada-Villa, I. Gasquet, V. Kovess, J. P. Lepine, M. C. Angermeyer, S. Bernert, G. de Girolamo, P. Morosini, et al., "Prevalence, Severity, and Unmet Need for Treatment of Mental Disorders in the World Health Organization World Mental Health Surveys," *Journal of the American Medical Association* 291, no. 21 (2004): 2581–90; R. C. Kessler, W. T. Chiu, O. Demler, K. R. Merikangas, and E. E. Walters, "Prevalence, Severity, and Comorbidity of 12-Month *DSM-IV* Disorders in the National Comorbidity Survey Replication," *Archives of General Psychiatry* 62, no. 6 (2005): 617–27.

5. M. Von Korff and D. Goldberg, "Improving Outcomes in Depression," *British Medical Journal,* 323, no. 7319 (2001): 948–49.

6. K. Rost, R. Smith, D. B. Matthews, and B. Guise, "The Deliberate Misdiagnosis of Major Depression in Primary Care," *Archives of Family Medicine* 3, no. 4 (1994): 333–37.

7. K. Kroenke, R. L. Spitzer, J. B. Williams, M. Linzer, S. R. Hahn, F. V. deGruy, III, and D. Brody, "Physical Symptoms in Primary Care: Predictors of Psychiatric Disorders and Functional Impairment," *Archives of Family Medicine* 3, no. 9 (1994): 774–79.

8. R. Kathol, S. Saravay, A. Lobo, and J. Ormel, "Epidemiologic Trends and Costs of Fragmentation," in *Medical Clinics of North America,* ed. F. Huyse and F. Stiefel (Philadelphia: Elsevier Saunders, 2006), 90: 549–72.

9. B. G. Druss, R. A. Rosenheck, and W. H. Sledge, "Health and Disability Costs of Depressive Illness in a Major U.S. Corporation," *American Journal of Psychiatry* 157, no. 8 (2000): 1274–78.

10. A. Gehi, D. Haas, S. Pipkin, and M. A. Whooley, "Depression and Medication Adherence in Outpatients with Coronary Heart Disease: Findings from the Heart and Soul Study," *Archives of Internal Medicine* 165, no. 21 (2005): 2508–13; W. Katon, C. R. Cantrell, M .C. Sokol, E. Chiao, and J. M. Gdovin, "Impact of Antidepressant Drug Adherence on Comorbid Medication Use and Resource Utilization," *Archives of Internal Medicine* 165, no. 21 (2005): 2497–2503.

11. R. A. Rosenheck, B. Druss, M. Stolar, D. Leslie, and W. Sledge, "Effect of Declining Mental Health Service Use on Employees of a Large Corporation," *Health Affairs (Project Hope)* 18, no. 5 (1999): 193–203.

12. A. M. Langlieb and J. P. Kahn, "How Much Does Quality Mental Health Care Profit Employers?" *Journal of Occupational and Environmental Medicine* 47, no. 11 (2005): 1099–1109.

13. R. Z. Goetzel, S. R. Long, R. J. Ozminkowski, K. Hawkins, S. Wang, and W. Lynch, "Health, Absence, Disability, and Presenteeism Cost Estimates of Certain Physical and Mental Health Conditions Affecting U.S. Employers," *Journal of Occupational and Environmental Medicine* 46, no. 4 (2004): 398–412.

14. R. G. Kathol, D. McAlpine, Y. Kishi, R. Spies, W. Meller, T. Bernhardt, S. Eisenberg, K. Folkert, and W. Gold, "General Medical and Pharmacy Claims Expenditures in Users of Behavioral Health Services," *Journal of General Internal Medicine* 20, no. 2 (2005): 160–67.

15. W. Katon, J. Unutzer, M. Y. Fan, J. W. Williams, Jr., M. Schoenbaum, E. H. Lin, and E. M. Hunkeler, "Cost-Effectiveness and Net Benefit of Enhanced Treatment of Depression

for Older Adults with Diabetes and Depression," *Diabetes Care* 29, no. 2 (2006): 265–70; E. M. Hunkeler, W. Katon, L. Tang, J. W. Williams, Jr., K. Kroenke, E. H. Lin, L. H. Harpole, P. Arean, S. Levine, L. M. Grypma et al., "Long Term Outcomes from the IMPACT Randomised Trial for Depressed Elderly Patients in Primary Care," *British Medical Journal* 332, no. 7536 (2006): 259–63.

16. S. Parthasarathy, J. Mertens, C. Moore, and C. Weisner, "Utilization and Cost Impact of Integrating Substance Abuse Treatment and Primary Care," *Medical Care* 41, no. 3 (2003): 357–67.

17. K. Rost, J. L. Smith, and M. Dickinson, "The Effect of Improving Primary Care Depression Management on Employee Absenteeism and Productivity: A Randomized Trial," *Medical Care* 42, no. 12 (2004): 1202–10. See also Katon et al., "Impact of Antidepressant Drug Adherence," and Goetzel et al., "Health, Absence, Disability, and Presenteeism."

18. S. Woolhandler, T. Campbell, and D. U. Himmelstein, "Health Care Administration in the United States and Canada: Micromanagement, Macro Costs," *International Journal of Health Services* 34, no. 1 (2004): 65–78.

CHAPTER 6

1. A. E. Perlman, *New York Times* (July 3, 1958). www.notdoneliving.net/quotes/quotes.cgi?topic=philosophy::positive (accessed January 5, 2007).

2. M. Dewan, "Are Psychiatrists Cost-Effective? An Analysis of Integrated versus Split Treatment," *American Journal of Psychiatry* 156, no. 2 (1999): 324–26.

3. B. W. Van Voorhees, N. Y. Wang, and D. E. Ford, "Managed Care Organizational Complexity and Access to High-Quality Mental Health Services: Perspective of U.S. Primary Care Physicians," *General Hospital Psychiatry* 25, no. 3 (2003): 149–57.

4. G. L. Larkin, C. A. Claassen, J. A. Emond, A. J. Pelletier, and C. A. Camargo, "Trends in U.S. Emergency Department Visits for Mental Health Conditions, 1992 to 2001," *Psychiatric Services* 56, no. 6 (2005): 671–77.

5. R. Z. Goetzel, S. R. Long, R. J. Ozminkowski, K. Hawkins, S. Wang, and W. Lynch, "Health, Absence, Disability, and Presenteeism Cost Estimates of Certain Physical and Mental Health Conditions Affecting U.S. Employers," *Journal of Occupational and Environmental Medicine* 46, no. 4 (2004): 398–412.

6. Y. Kishi and R. G. Kathol, "Integrating Medical and Psychiatric Treatment in an Inpatient Medical Setting: The Type IV Program," *Psychosomatics* 40, no. 4 (1999): 345–55.

7. R. Kathol, S. Saravay, A. Lobo, and J. Ormel, "Epidemiologic Trends and Costs of Fragmentation," in *Medical Clinics of North America,* ed. F. Huyse and F. Stiefel (Philadelphia: Elsivier Saunders, 2006) 90:549–72.

CHAPTER 7

1. H. D. Thoreau, "Conclusion to Walden," in *Walden* (Boston: Ticknor and Fields, 1854).

2. R. Kathol and A. Stoudemire, "Strategic Integration of Inpatient and Outpatient Medical-Psychiatry Services," in *The Textbook of Consultation-Liaison Psychiatry* (2nd ed.), ed. M. G. Wise and J. R. Rundell (Washington, DC: APPI Press, 2002), 995–1014.

3. W. Katon, J. Unutzer, M. Y. Fan, J. W. Williams, Jr., M. Schoenbaum, E. H. Lin, and E. M. Hunkeler, "Cost-Effectiveness and Net Benefit of Enhanced Treatment of Depression for Older Adults with Diabetes and Depression," *Diabetes Care* 29, no. 2 (2006): 265–70.

4. F. Stiefel, F. Huyse, W. Söllner, J. P. J. Slaets, J. S. Lyons, C. H. M. Latour, N. van der Wal, and P. de Jonge, "Operationalizing Integrated Care on a Clinical Level: The

INTERMED Project," in *Medical Clinics of North America,* ed. F. Huyse and F. Stiefel (New York: Elsivier, 2006), 90:713–58.

5. F. Huyse, F. Stiefel, and P.D. Jonge, "Identifiers or 'Red Flag' of Complexity and Need for Integrated Care," in *Medical Clinics of North America,* ed. F. Huyse and F. Stiefel (New York: Elsevier, 2006), 90:703–12.

6. G.L. Larkin, C.A. Claassen, J.A. Emond, A.J. Pelletier, and C.A. Camargo, "Trends in U.S. Emergency Department Visits for Mental Health Conditions, 1992 to 2001," *Psychiatric Services* 56, no. 6 (2005): 671–77.

7. National Association of State Mental Health Program Directors, "State Psychiatric Hospitals: 2004," *NASMHDP Research Institute, Inc.* (September 2005), http://www.nri-inc.org/Profiles04/2004StateHospital.pdf (last accessed December 14, 2006).

8. R.A. Rosenblatt, C.H. Andrilla, T. Curtin, and L.G. Hart, "Shortages of Medical Personnel at Community Health Centers: Implications for Planned Expansion," *Journal of the American Medical Association* 295, no. 9 (2006): 1042–49.

CHAPTER 8

1. Attributed to Walt Disney.

CHAPTER 9

1. Attributed to Abraham Lincoln.

2. D. Sacher, *Mental Health: A Report of the Surgeon General,* United States Department of Health and Human Services. (accessed December 16, 2006). http://www.surgeongeneral.gov/library/mentalhealth/home.html

3. President's New Freedom Commission on Mental Health, *Achieving the Promise: Transforming Mental Health Care in America* (Rockville, MD: Substance Abuse and Mental Health Services Administration, 2003; accessed December 16, 2006). http://www.mentalhealthcommission.gov/reports/FinalReport/toc.html

4. Institute of Medicine. *Improving the Quality of Health Care for Mental and Substance-Use Conditions: Quality Chasm Series* (Washington: National Academies Press, 2005); Institute of Medicine. *Crossing the Quality Chasm: A New Health System for the 21st Century.* (Washington, DC: National Academies Press, 2001).

5. Institute of Medicine. *Improving the Quality of Health Care,* "Recommendation 5-2":16–17.

6. Ibid.

7. G.L. Larkin, C.A. Claassen, J.A. Emond, A.J. Pelletier, and C.A. Camargo, "Trends in U.S. Emergency Department Visits for Mental Health Conditions, 1992 to 2001," *Psychiatric Services* 56, no. 6 (2005): 671–77.

8. D.C. Lewis, "Alcohol Screening Fulfills Important Duty to Patients," *American Medical News* (March 6, 2006; accessed December 16, 2006). http://198.178.213.111/amednews/2006/03/06/prcb0306.html

9. M.F. Fleming, M.P. Mundt, M.T. French, L.B. Manwell, E.A. Stauffacher, and K.L. Barry, "Brief Physician Advice for Problem Drinkers: Long-Term Efficacy and Benefit-Cost Analysis," *Alcoholism, Clinical and Experimental Research* 26, no. 1 (2002): 36–43.

10. M.D. Feldman, *Playing Sick?: Untangling the Web of Munchausen Syndrome, Munchausen by Proxy, Malingering, and Factitious Disorder* (New York: Brunner-Routledge, 2004).

11. B. Truman and E. W. Ely, "Monitoring Delirium in Critically Ill Patients: Using the Confusion Assessment Method for the Intensive Care Unit," *Critical Care Nurse* 23, no. 2 (2003): 25–36.

12. P. Earley, *Crazy: A Father's Search through America's Mental Health Madness* (New York: Putnam, 2006).

INDEX

About the Authors

ROGER KATHOL, M.D. is an Adjunct Professor of Internal Medicine and Psychiatry at the University of Minnesota, and also President of an integrated health care consulting company, Cartesian Solutions Inc. He is past President of the American Academy of Clinical Psychiatry as well as the Academy of Psychosomatic Medicine. Kathol is also Founding President of the Association of Medicine and Psychiatry.

SUZANNE GATTEAU is a freelance writer.